BODY [illegible]se

your guide to growing up

KAREN BRYANT-MOLE

About this book

This book has been written to prepare children for the physical and emotional changes that occur as they grow up. It takes a comprehensive look at body changes and changes in personal relationships.

The book also discusses sexual intercourse, reproduction and contraception. It presents this as information which will be needed in the future and it stresses the importance of responsibility, self-respect and choice.

There is information, too, about smoking, drugs and alcohol. Part of growing up involves making decisions on your own. Reasoned decisions can only be made if you have the necessary information.

Many parents and teachers find it difficult to talk to children about growing up. Often, this is because they feel embarrassed. Sometimes, it is because they don't know where to start. This book is intended to solve those problems.

Children should be encouraged to discuss what they read here. It is important that children know that there is someone they can talk to about growing up.

First published in 1997 by
Health Education Authority
Hamilton House
Mabledon Place
London WC1H 9TX, UK

British Library Cataloguing in Publication Data
A CIP catalogue record for this book is available from the British Library

ISBN 1 85448 957 7

Design: Amanda Hawkes
Cover illustration: Ann Johns
Text illustrations: Helen Herbert, Annabel Milne
Text cartoons: Ann Johns
Text photographs: Colin Taylor Productions except page 4 which is reproduced with the permission of Sally and Richard Greenhill; pages 13, 27 and 40 which are reproduced with the permission of Bubbles Photo Library; pages 31 and 32 which are reproduced with the permission of the Science Photo Library; and page 34 which is reproduced with the permission of Zefa Pictures.

Printed in Great Britain.

Contents

Some of the more difficult words are explained in the glossary.

Puberty

Do you know what the weather will be like next month? Do you know what you will be eating for dinner next year? Lots of things about life are uncertain. But one thing is certain and that is that all children grow up.

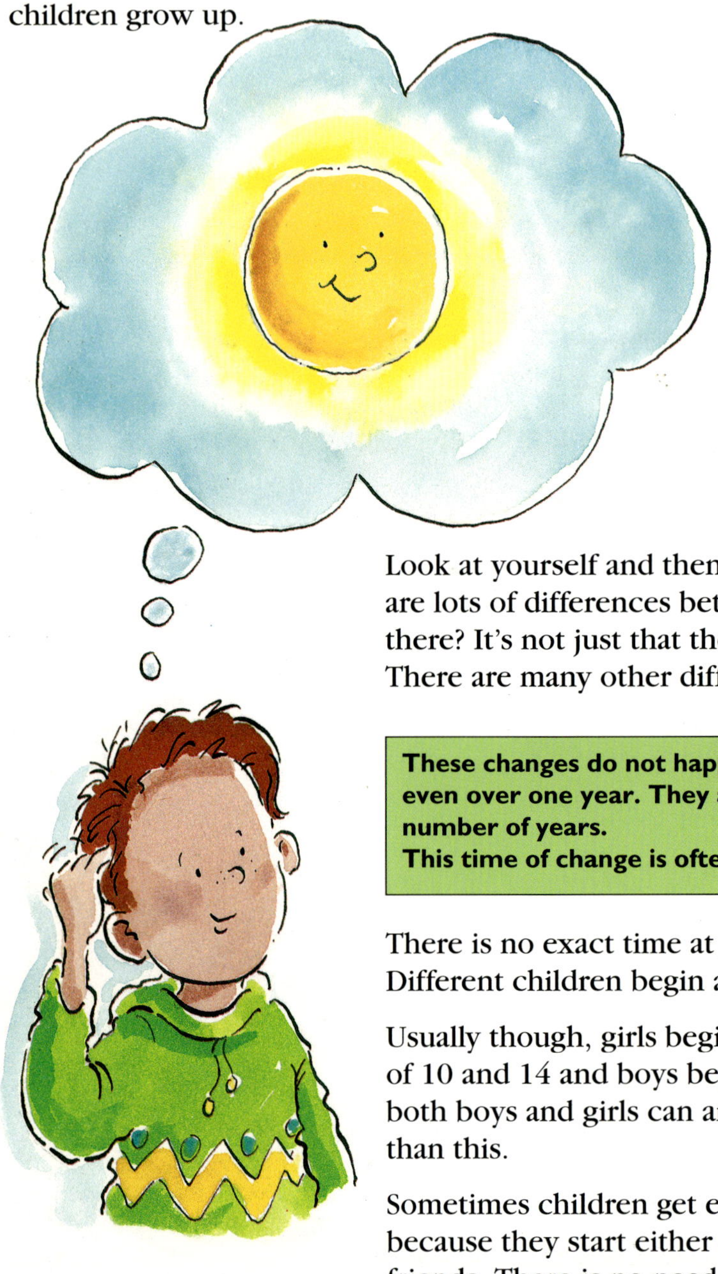

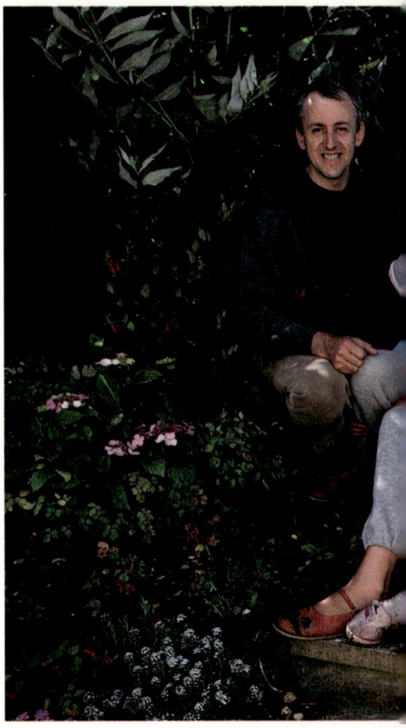

Look at yourself and then look at a grown-up. There are lots of differences between the two of you, aren't there? It's not just that the grown-up is taller than you. There are many other differences to notice, too.

These changes do not happen to your body overnight or even over one year. They are usually spread out over a number of years.
This time of change is often called 'puberty'.

There is no exact time at which puberty begins. Different children begin at different times.

Usually though, girls begin puberty between the ages of 10 and 14 and boys begin between 11 and 15. But both boys and girls can and do start earlier or later than this.

Sometimes children get embarrassed or worried because they start either earlier or later than their friends. There is no need to feel like this. There is nothing wrong with starting early or late. Your body will start to change when it is ready but if you are worried, talk to your parents or school nurse.

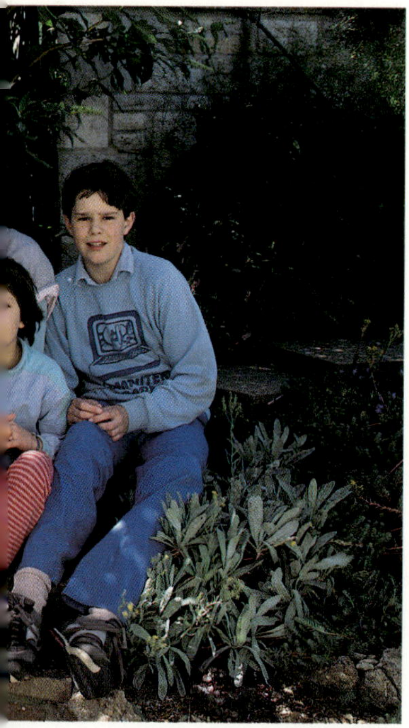

HOW DOES PUBERTY START?

All this changing and growing is controlled by something called your **hormones**.

Hormones are special chemicals made by your body.

These chemicals send messages to the various parts of your body and tell them to get into action and start to grow and develop.

WILL I KNOW WHEN PUBERTY HAS STARTED?

For many children the first sign of puberty is that they do a lot of growing in a short time. Clothes that used to fit are suddenly too small. Other children find that it is one of the other body changes that let them know that puberty is beginning. We'll look at some of those changes on the next page.

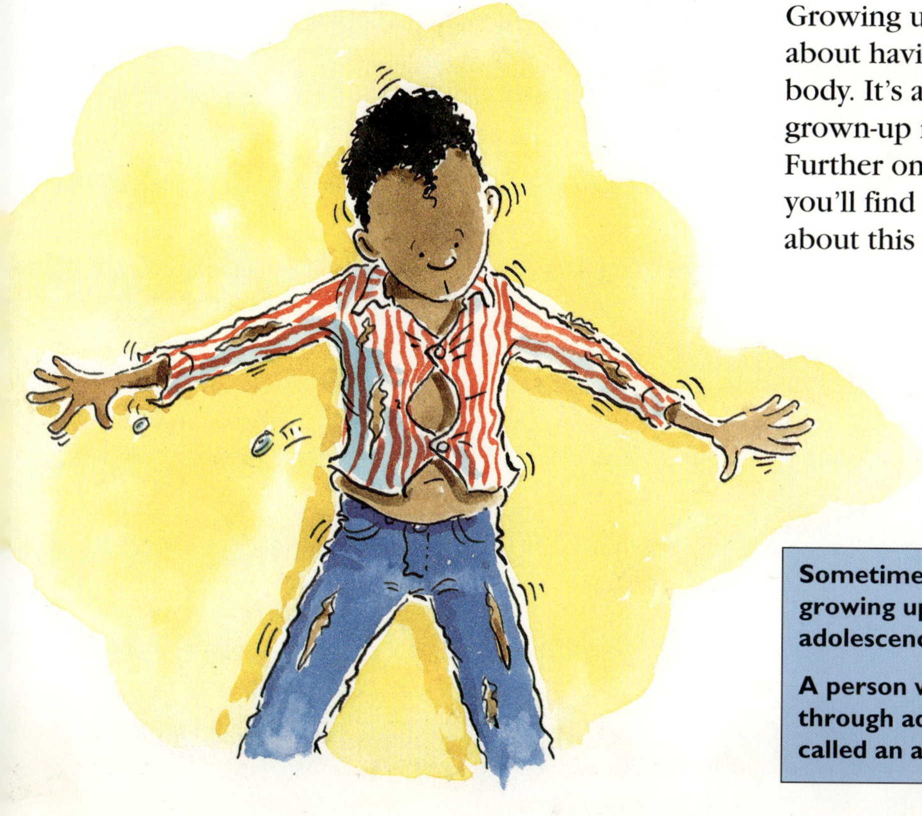

Growing up isn't just about having a grown-up body. It's about having a grown-up mind as well. Further on in the book you'll find out a bit more about this too.

Sometimes this time of growing up is called adolescence.

A person who is going through adolescence is called an adolescent.

Body changes

These pictures of children and adults show you most of the important changes that will happen to your body during puberty. But, remember, you won't look like the child one day and the adult the next. There is a long, in-between time during which your body will be gradually changing from one to the other.

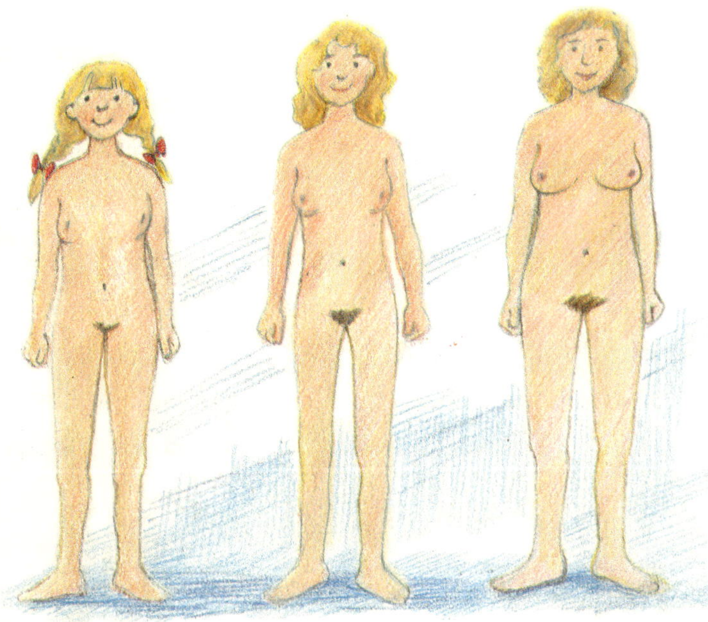

GIRLS

Your breasts will start to develop. Some girls find that this is the first sign of puberty.

You will grow body hair. Hair grows under your arms. It also grows between your legs and into a triangle shape. This hair is called pubic hair.

Your hips will get wider.

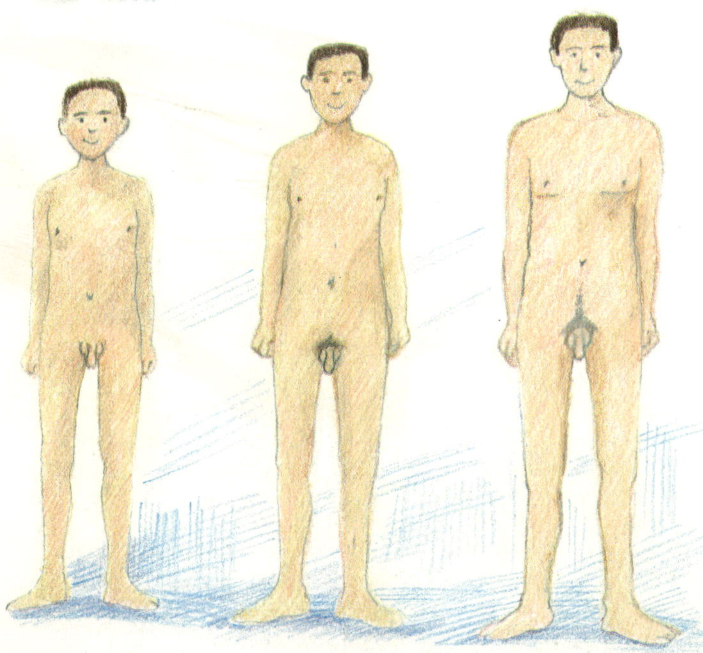

BOYS

The Adam's apple in your throat will get bigger and your voice will get deeper. This is known as your voice 'breaking'.

Your shoulders and your chest will probably get wider.

You too will grow body hair. It will grow under your arms, between your legs and around the bottom of your penis and on your testes. You will also start to grow hair on your face.

Your penis and testes will gradually get bigger.

Children start puberty at different times and develop at different rates. This means that at any one time you and your friends will probably all have very different-looking bodies.

Even when puberty has come to an end and you all have your grown-up bodies you are still going to look very different to one another. Look at the grown-ups you know and see how different they are!

Sometimes, children feel uncomfortable in their growing bodies. Your arms and legs or hands and feet might grow faster than the rest of your body and this could make you feel clumsy or awkward.

This feeling doesn't usually last long.

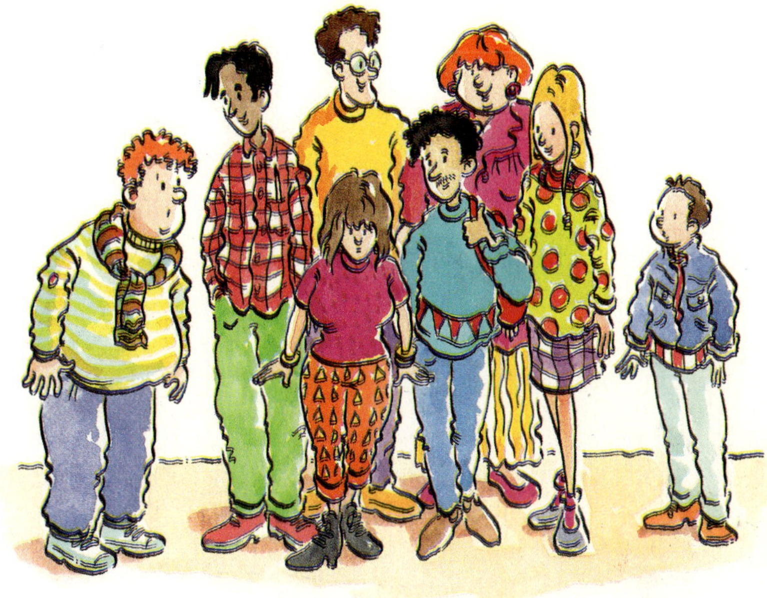

LIKING YOUR NEW BODY

Sometimes, children find learning to like their bodies difficult. It isn't helped by some of the pictures we see in adverts and in magazines.

Often these pictures seem to be saying that if you want to be happy and successful, you have to be a particular shape. This is completely untrue.

What you are like as a person is more important than the shape of your body.

Think of all the people you know who don't fit this idea of the 'right' shape but who are happy and successful.

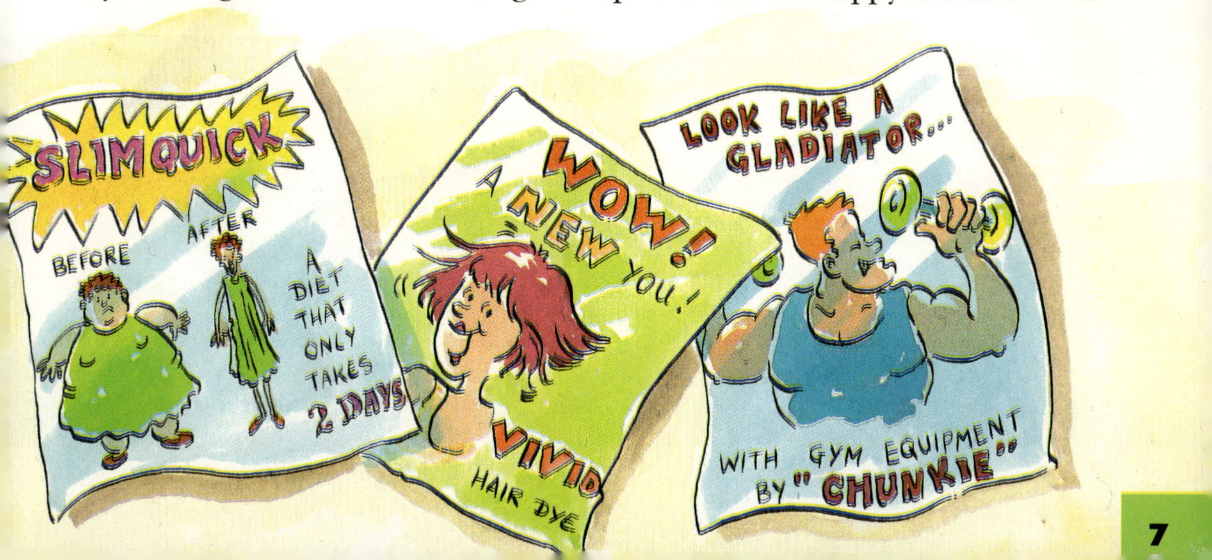
SLIMQUICK
BEFORE
AFTER
A DIET THAT ONLY TAKES 2 DAYS
WOW!
A NEW YOU!
VIVID
HAIR DYE
LOOK LIKE A GLADIATOR...
WITH GYM EQUIPMENT BY "CHUNKIE"

Body hair

The first body hair to start growing is usually your pubic hair.

At first there will be just a few soft hairs. You will gradually grow more and they will become thicker and darker as you progress through puberty.

Don't worry if your pubic hair feels different or is a different colour to the hair on your head. This often happens. And even if you have completely straight hair on your head, your pubic hair is quite likely to end up curly.

Pubic hair may start growing anywhere from the navel, or tummy button, downwards.

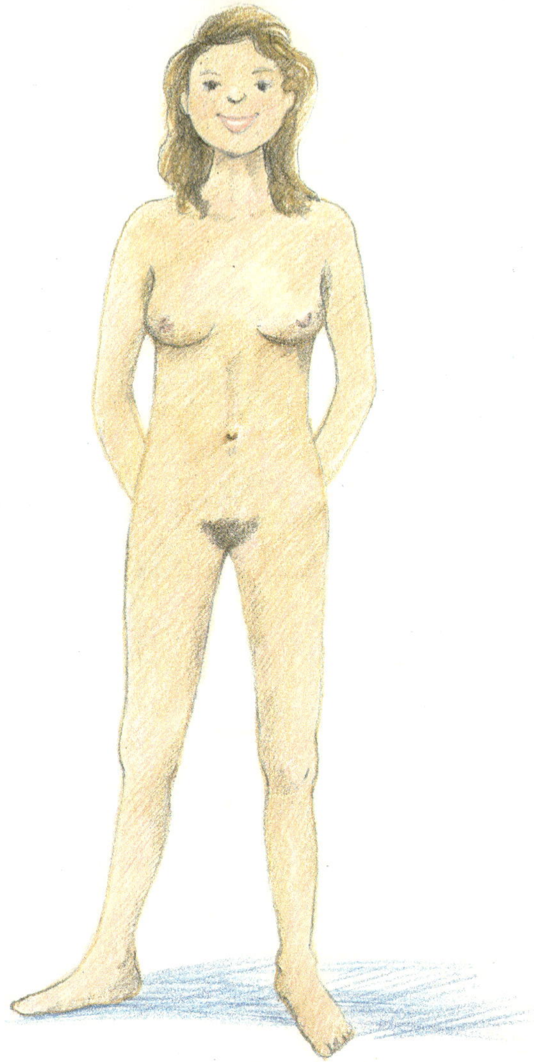

Hair usually starts to grow under your arms a year or so after your pubic hair has begun to grow. But don't worry if it starts growing before your pubic hair.

Many girls find that the hair on their upper lip gets slightly darker during puberty.

The hair on your arms and legs will probably get darker too as you grow up.

Later on in puberty many boys start to grow hair on their chests. Some boys end up with a lot while others have very little.

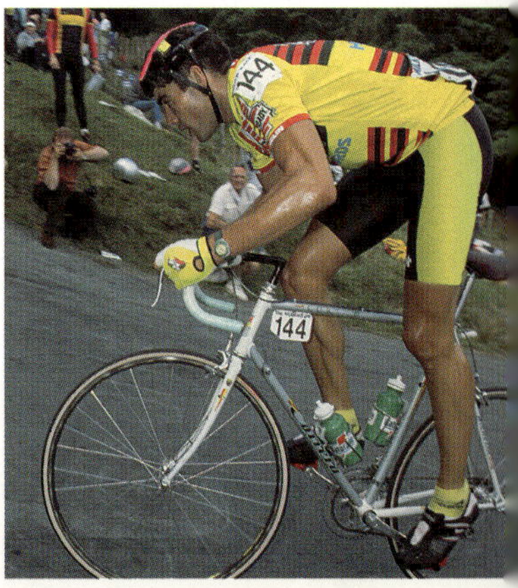

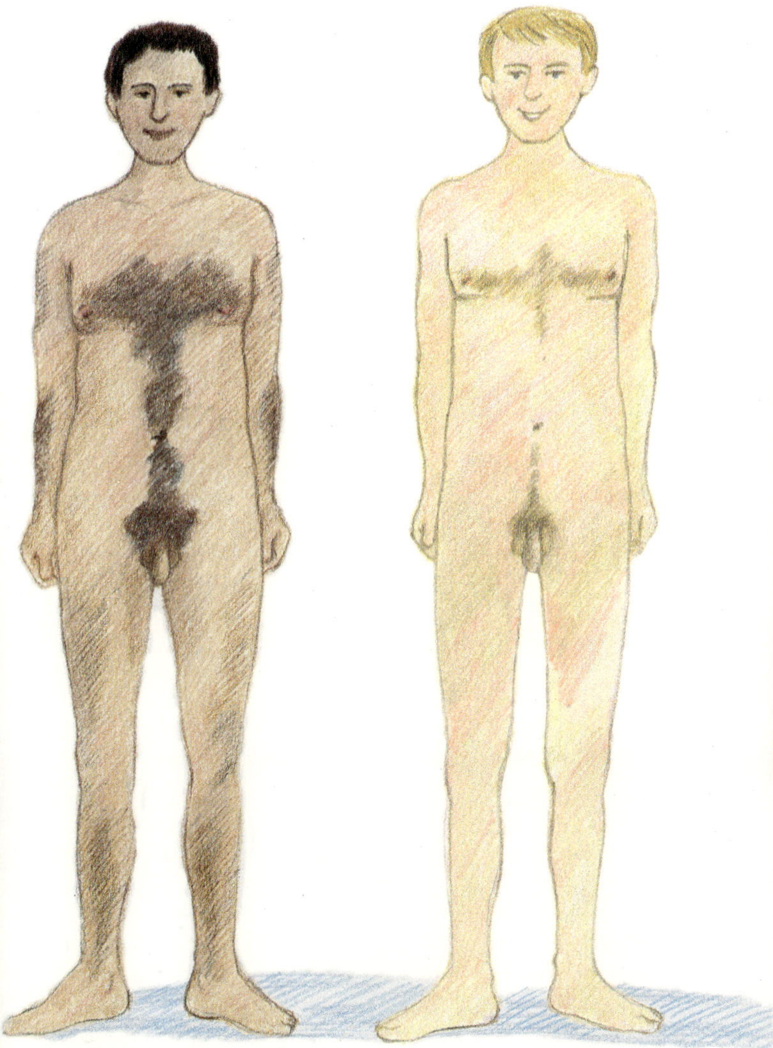

It is not unusual to find dark hairs growing on your shoulders, the back of your hands and sometimes your feet.

Some people decide to remove some of their body hair either because they think it looks better or because they take part in sports.

But you don't have to if you don't want to.

If you decide to remove it, you can either shave it or use a special hair-removing cream.

FACIAL HAIR

One of the last body changes to happen to boys is that hair starts to grow on your face.

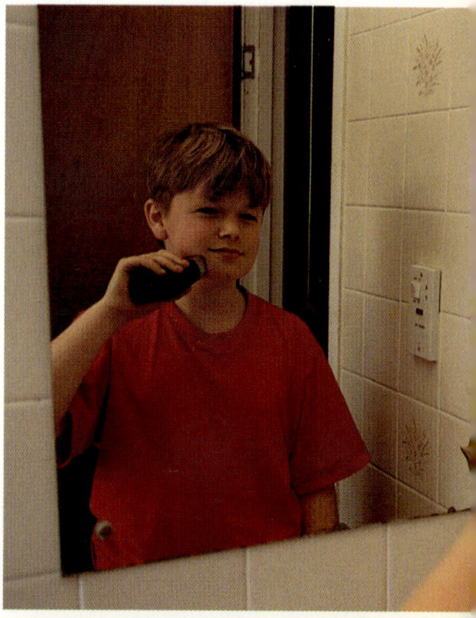

At first there will just be a fine growth of darker hair on your upper lip. Eventually this hair will become thicker and you may want to shave it.

You can do this with an electric shaver or a hand razor that you use with foam and warm water.

When you first begin shaving you will not need to shave every day. You may eventually need to shave regularly unless you want to grow a beard or moustache.

Skin

During puberty your body starts to make more of an oily substance called sebum.

We all need sebum to stop our skin and hair drying out but if you are producing a lot of sebum you may find that your hair is greasier than usual and that spots start appearing, especially on your face, neck, chest and back.

You might find that keeping your skin as clear of sebum as possible, by washing thoroughly at least once a day, helps to reduce the number of spots you have.

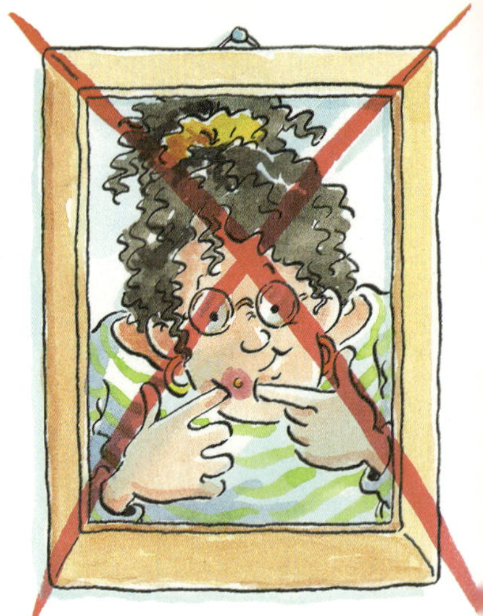

Try not to squeeze spots. Picking spots makes them worse and they then take much longer to clear up and may even leave small scars.

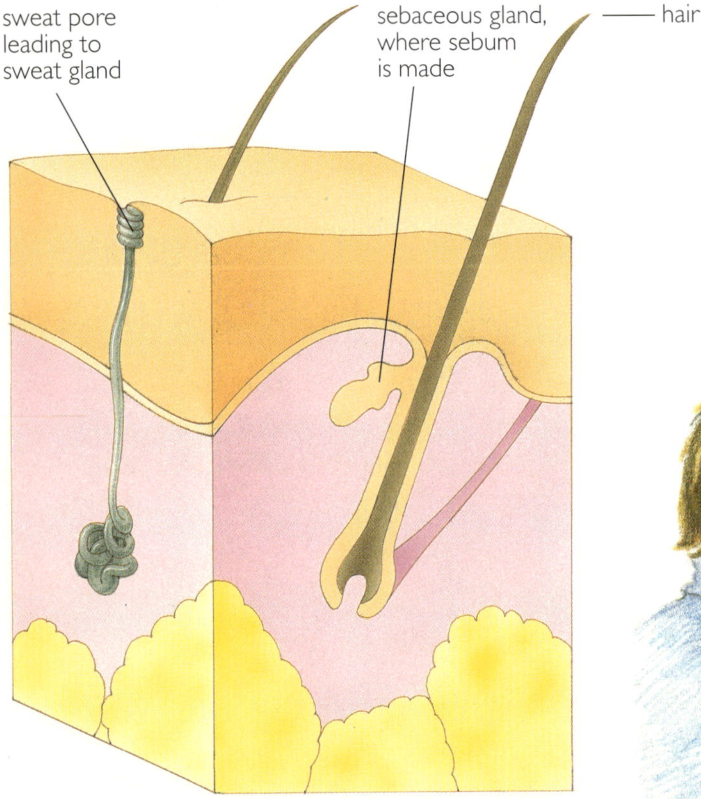

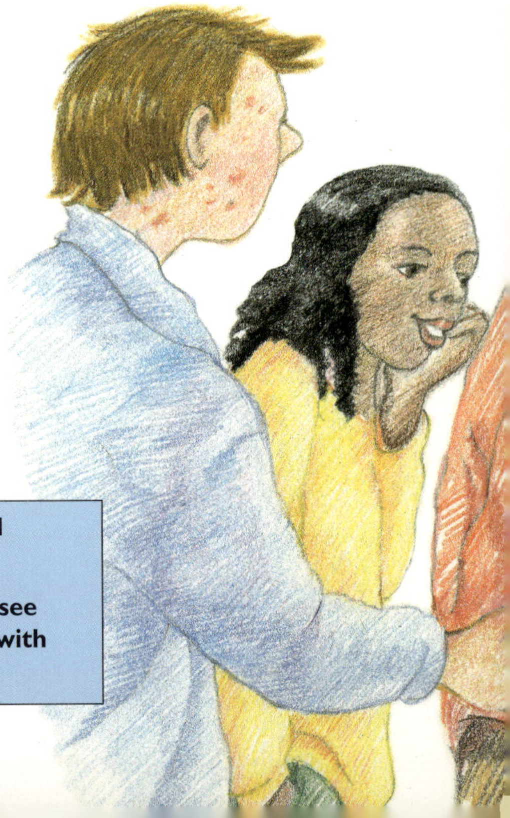

For some people, though, spots can become a real problem.

If your spots become a problem, you could go and see your doctor who will probably be able to help you with special creams or tablets.

There are two things to remember about spots.

One – there is more to you than your spots. Your skin is not you. You, as a person, are far more important than your skin.

Two – spots and greasy hair are things that almost all of us grow out of. Your hormones have made your body produce this extra sebum. When your hormones settle down your body will stop producing too much sebum.

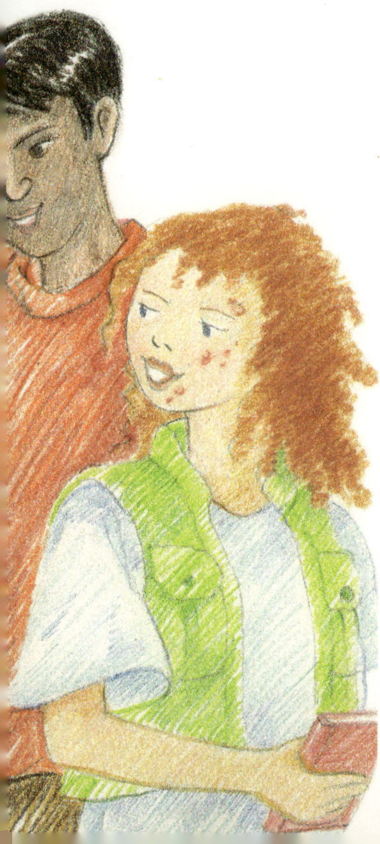

SWEAT

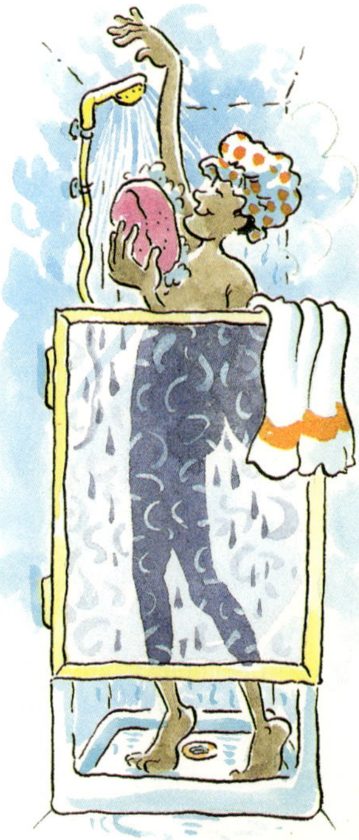

As you go through puberty, you will find that your body starts to make more sweat.

You will probably notice it most under your arms and between your legs.

Old sweat does not smell very nice so it is important that you wash yourself well every day.

Clothes that come into contact with sweat will soak up the sweat and start to smell too.

So, put your clean body into clean clothes.

Sometimes people are worried about sweating or are embarrassed by damp patches under their arms.

Unfortunately, worrying about sweating usually makes you sweat more.

Sweating is perfectly normal. We all do it. But, if you choose to, you can use an anti-perspirant or a deodorant under your arms and this will probably help.

Anti-perspirants make you sweat less and deodorants stop sweat smelling.

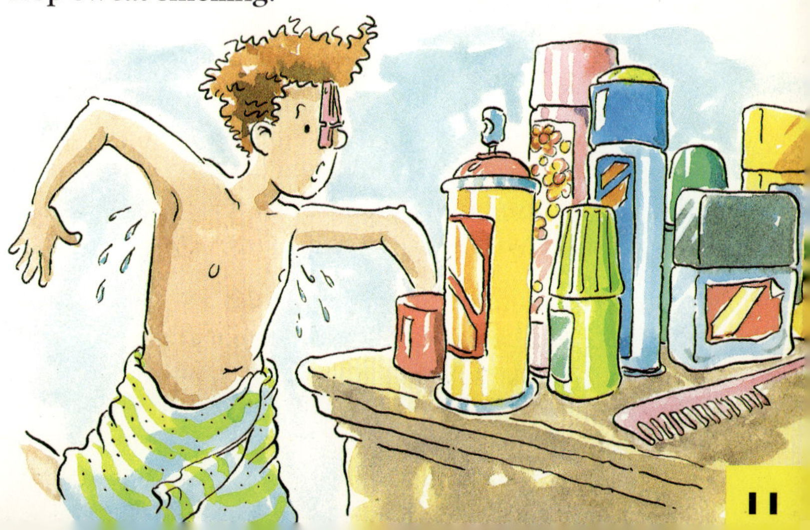

Breasts

Boys! This page is for you, too. Even though your breasts won't grow, it is important to know about this and all the other body changes that are happening to girls. It is just as important for girls to understand boys' bodies too.

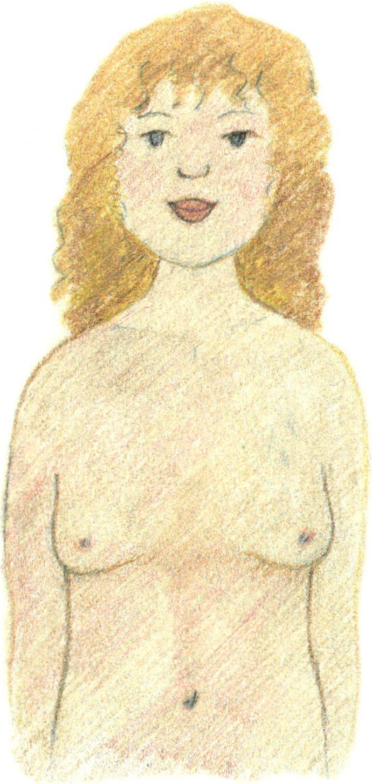

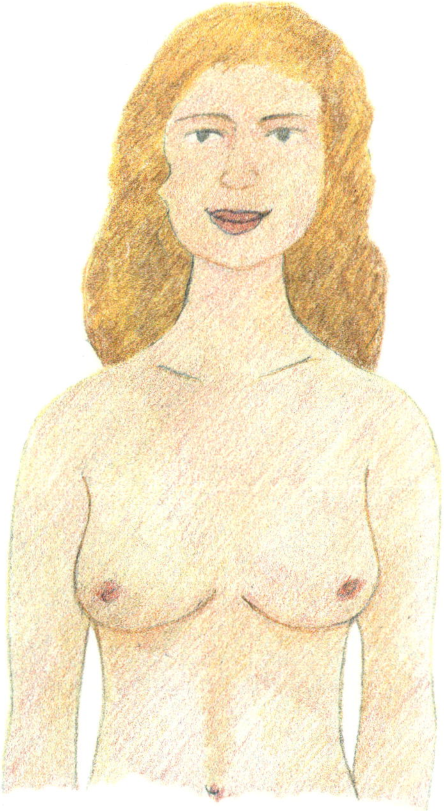

Usually, the first stage of the growth of a girl's breasts is when a small amount of fatty tissue begins to form underneath your nipple and areola. (Your areola is the coloured circle around your nipple.)

Some girls find that their breasts sometimes feel sore and tender. Although this might be a bit painful at times, it isn't anything to worry about.

As you go through puberty, your breasts will continue to develop and become fuller and more rounded. The nipple and areola will probably get bigger and turn a darker colour.

Sometimes boys find that they get some swelling around their breasts too. There is nothing wrong with this. It is just your hormones again. The swelling will disappear as puberty goes on.

Sometimes, girls worry because one breast seems to be growing faster than the other. This is perfectly normal.

Even when your breasts have stopped growing, you will probably find that they are not exactly the same size.

Breasts and nipples come in all shapes and sizes. Sometimes, one or both nipples go inwards instead of sticking out. These are called inverted nipples. They don't usually cause any problems, though.

Sometimes, girls wish that their breasts were smaller or larger than they actually are but there are no exercises or diets that will alter the size of your breasts.

It doesn't really matter what size your breasts are and all sizes work equally well for feeding babies.

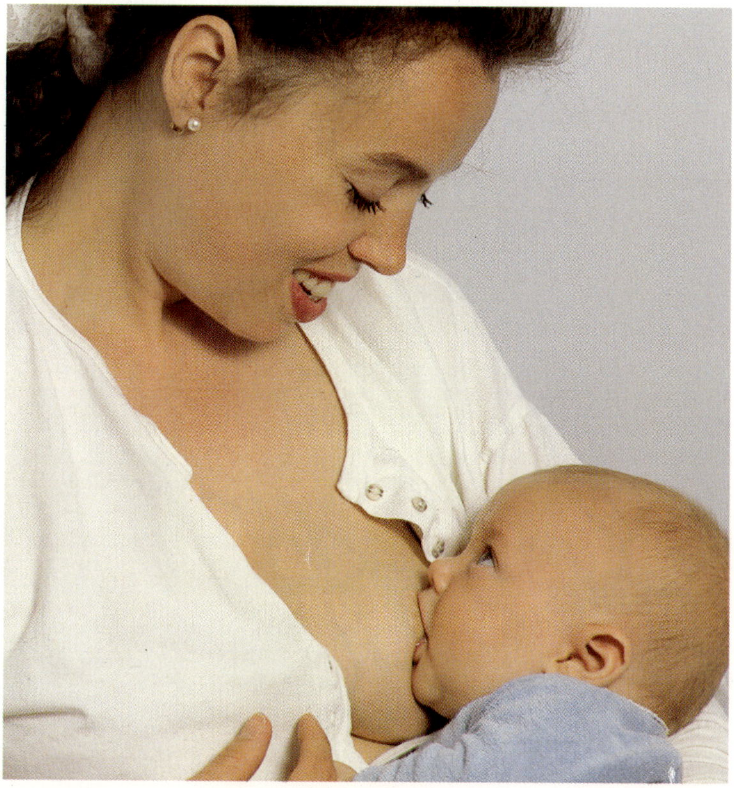

When a woman has a baby her body will start to produce milk. The baby will be able to suck the milk through tiny holes in her nipples.

WEARING A BRA

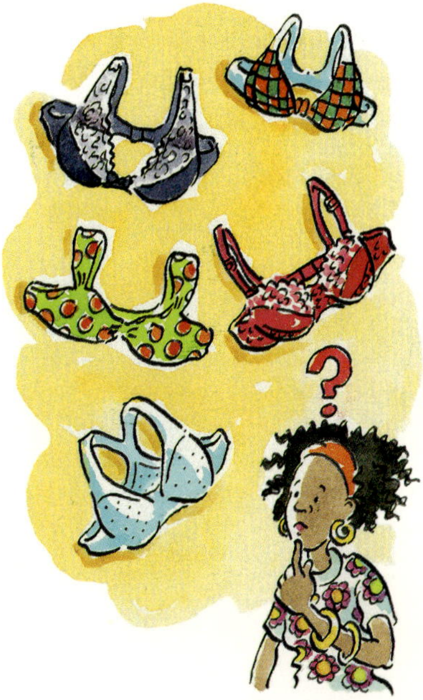

Most girls choose to wear a bra. If you do, make sure that you buy a bra that fits you well. Many shops let you try them on before you buy. Don't forget that as your breasts grow and change shape you will probably need to change the size of your bra.

If you don't want to wear a bra you don't have to, although some girls find running or playing sport uncomfortable if they don't wear a bra. If you have large breasts it is probably a good idea, as a bra will give your breasts some support.

Boys

SCROTUM This is the bag of skin behind your penis.

Inside your scrotum are your two testes. These are small and egg-shaped.

PENIS Your penis is the part of your body that you use when you go for a wee. Families often have their own names for this part of your body.

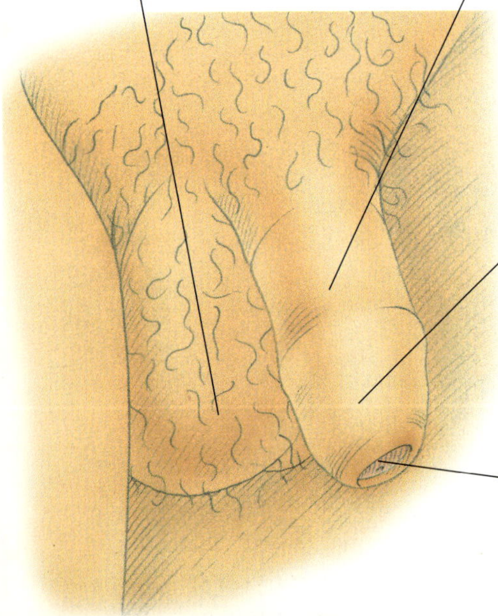

FORESKIN Your penis may have a loose fold of skin at the end of it. This is your foreskin. It protects the end of your penis.

Some boys have their foreskin removed.
This is called circumcision.

GLANS This is the proper name for the end of your penis.

The pictures show an adult male's genitals, so don't worry if yours don't look exactly the same.

During puberty, your penis and testes will get bigger. These parts of your body are known as your genitals.

Your testes usually start growing first. They produce sperm, which are the man's part of making a baby. You will probably find that the testis on the left hangs down lower than the one on the right.

Your penis will probably begin to grow about a year after your testes, although it could be sooner or later than this. Lots of boys worry about the size of their penis. There is no need to. A long penis is no better or worse than a short one.

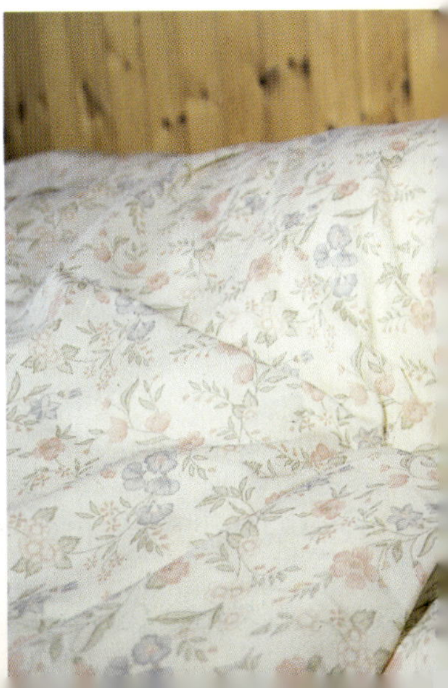

ERECTIONS

An erection is when the penis becomes hard, rather than soft, and much bigger. Instead of hanging down, it points upwards and away from the body. This is because the body has pumped extra blood into the penis.

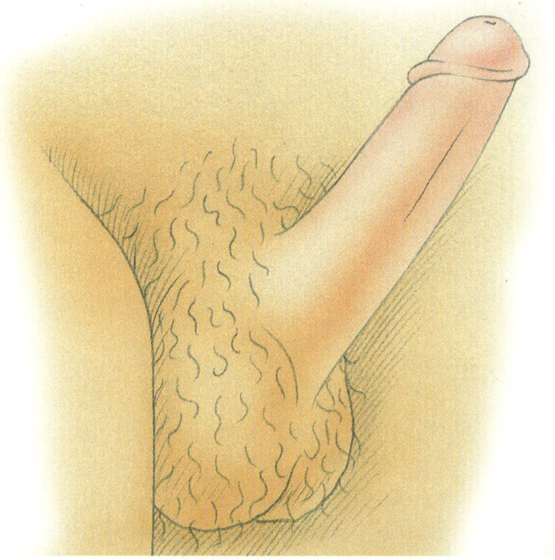

Many boys have erections throughout their childhood.

During puberty you will probably find that you get more erections. Sometimes, boys get an erection by touching their penises. Often, erections just happen all by themselves. These are called spontaneous erections.

Boys are sometimes embarrassed by them but it is worth remembering that they probably aren't as noticeable as you think they are. Boys usually soon get used to them.

WET DREAMS

Most boys have wet dreams during puberty. A wet dream means that you have an erection while you are asleep and semen squirts out of the end of your penis.

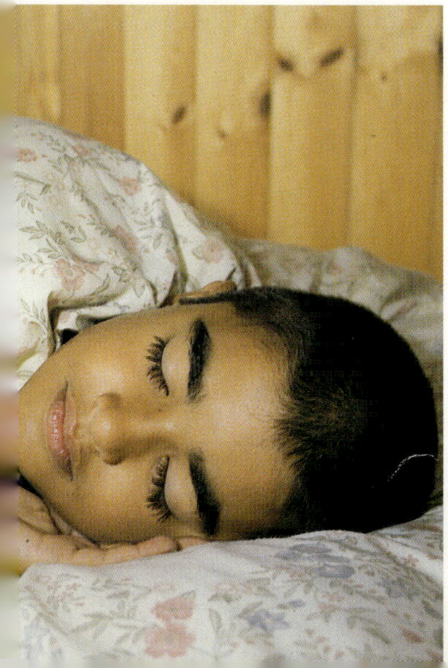

You may wake up and find a small amount of sticky liquid in the bed. This is the semen. Semen is a mixture of sperm and fluid for the sperm to swim in. When semen squirts out of the end of your penis this is called ejaculation.

Wet dreams are nothing to worry about. They are a healthy sign that you are growing up and your body is working well. Some boys have their first ejaculation in their sleep. Others have their first ejaculation after getting an erection by touching or rubbing their penises.

People sometimes rub their genitals because it gives them a nice feeling. This is called masturbating.

Girls

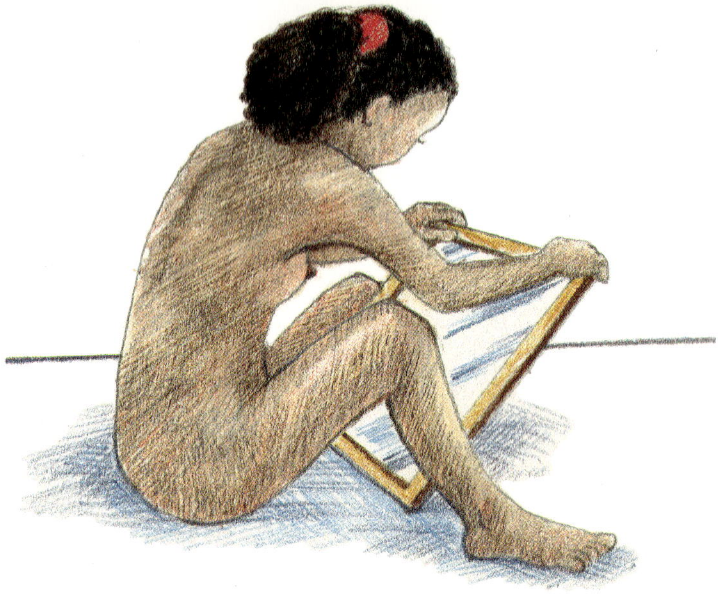

The parts of a girl's body that are between your legs are called your genitals.

Unlike boys, it is rather hard for you, as girls, to see your own genitals.

If you are not sure where all the parts mentioned on this page are, you might find it helpful to sit on the floor and use a mirror to look at your genitals.

Don't worry if your genitals don't look exactly like those in the drawing.

Everyone's genitals are a different size and shape.

LABIA
These are the parts of your genitals that are the easiest to see.

You have two plump, soft lips called the outer labia and inside these are two thinner folds of skin called the inner labia.

URINARY OPENING
This is the small hole that your wee, or urine, comes through.

Although you probably won't be able to see it, it is between your clitoris and your vaginal opening.

VAGINAL OPENING
In between your labia you will be able to see or feel an opening. This is the entrance to your vagina.

CLITORIS Your clitoris is very tiny. You might be able to feel it as a small lump where the inner labia join, towards the front of your body.

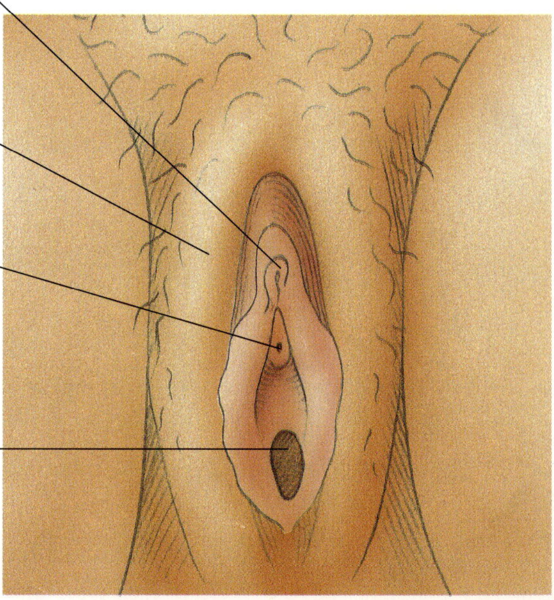

Some of the changes that happen to a girl during puberty are to do with parts of your body that can't be seen from the outside. The easiest way to show these parts of your body is to use a drawing called a cross-section.

A cross-section shows you the inside of something in the same way that you can see the inside of an apple if it is cut in two.

UTERUS This is sometimes called your womb. If you were having a baby, this is where the baby would grow. It is hollow and made of muscle.

OVARIES This is where tiny egg cells, called ova, are stored. They are the woman's part of making a baby. One egg cell is called an ovum.

FALLOPIAN OR UTERINE TUBES These thin, hollow tubes start from near each of the ovaries and lead to the uterus.

VAGINA Your vagina is tube-shaped and goes upwards inside your body.

CERVIX The cervix is sometimes called the neck of the womb. It is found at the top of your vagina.

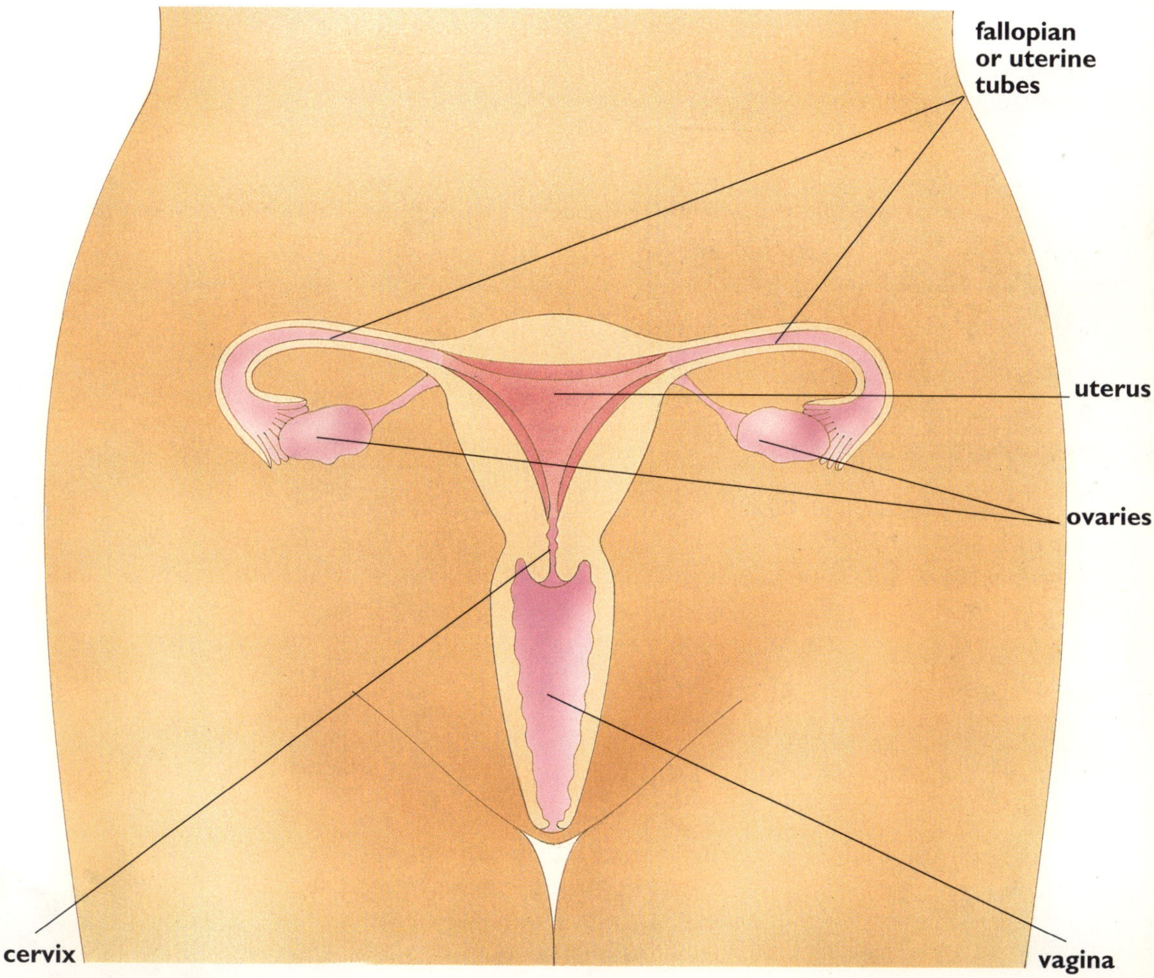

Periods

At some point during puberty, girls start to have periods.

Many girls find that their periods start a year or so after their breasts have begun to develop, but they can start earlier or later than this.

Before they begin their periods many girls start producing a clear or cream-coloured fluid. This is normal. It helps protect against germs and keeps the vagina clean. It is sometimes called vaginal fluid.

WHERE DOES THE BLOOD COME FROM?

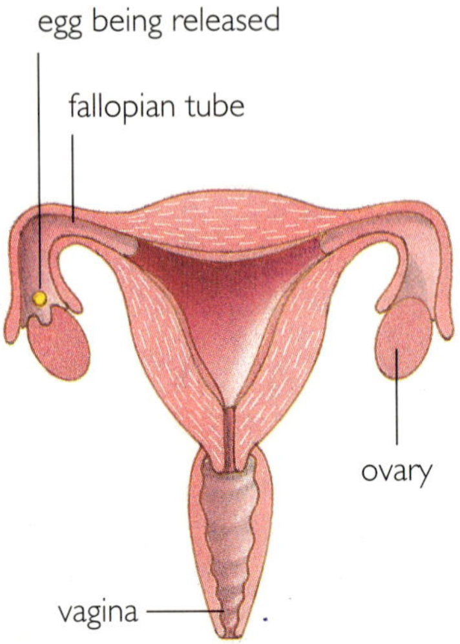

During puberty your body starts to release the egg cells, or ova, that are stored in your ovaries. These egg cells are the woman's part of making a baby.

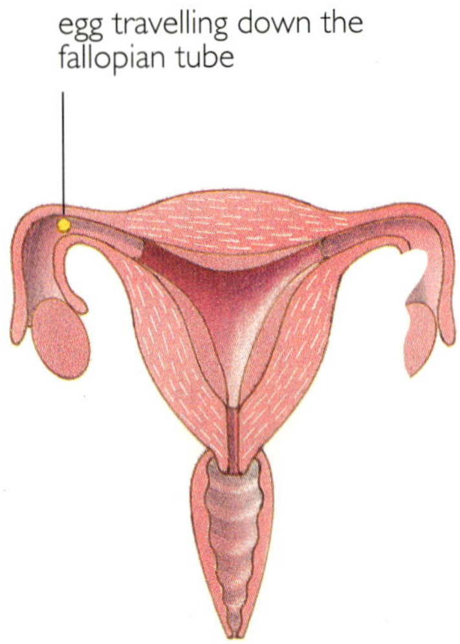

About once a month an egg travels down one of your fallopian tubes. At the same time, the lining of the uterus grows thick and spongy with extra blood vessels.

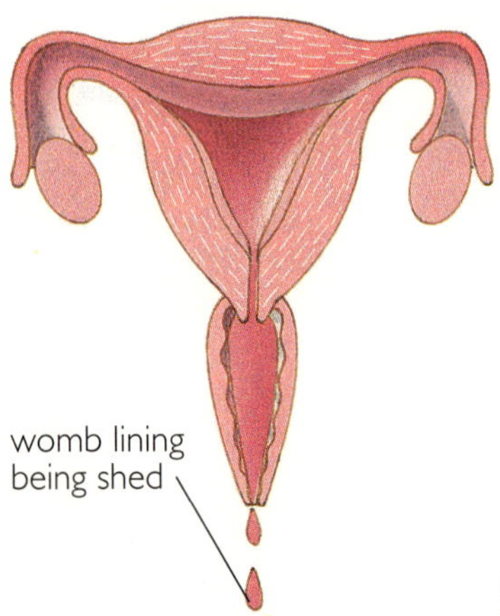

If the egg is not going to become a baby that month, the lining of the uterus is shed, or comes away, and blood comes out slowly through the vagina over a few days.

WHAT IS A PERIOD?

A period is when a small amount of blood passes out through a girl's vagina.

This happens about once a month and usually lasts between three and seven days.

After your first period, the next may not happen for several weeks. This is quite usual. As you get older, they will probably settle down into more of a pattern.

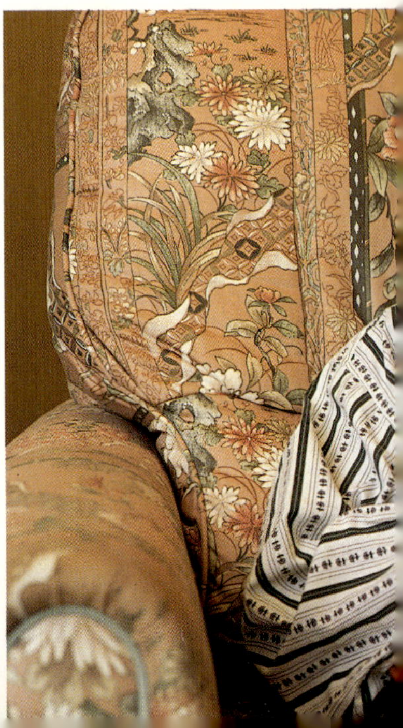

WHAT HAPPENS TO THE BLOOD?

You can buy special pads called sanitary towels. These go in your knickers and soak up the blood as it comes out of your vagina. Sanitary towels usually have a sticky strip on the bottom to keep them in place.

Most girls start by using sanitary towels but, later, some may prefer to use tampons. You can use whichever you find easier and more comfortable.

Tampons go inside your vagina and soak up the blood as it leaves the uterus. They come in different sizes. You will probably need a small size at first. Remember to read the instructions inside the box.

Towels and tampons both need to be changed regularly. If you use tampons, make sure you remove the last tampon at the end of each period. If it is left in your vagina, it may become infected.

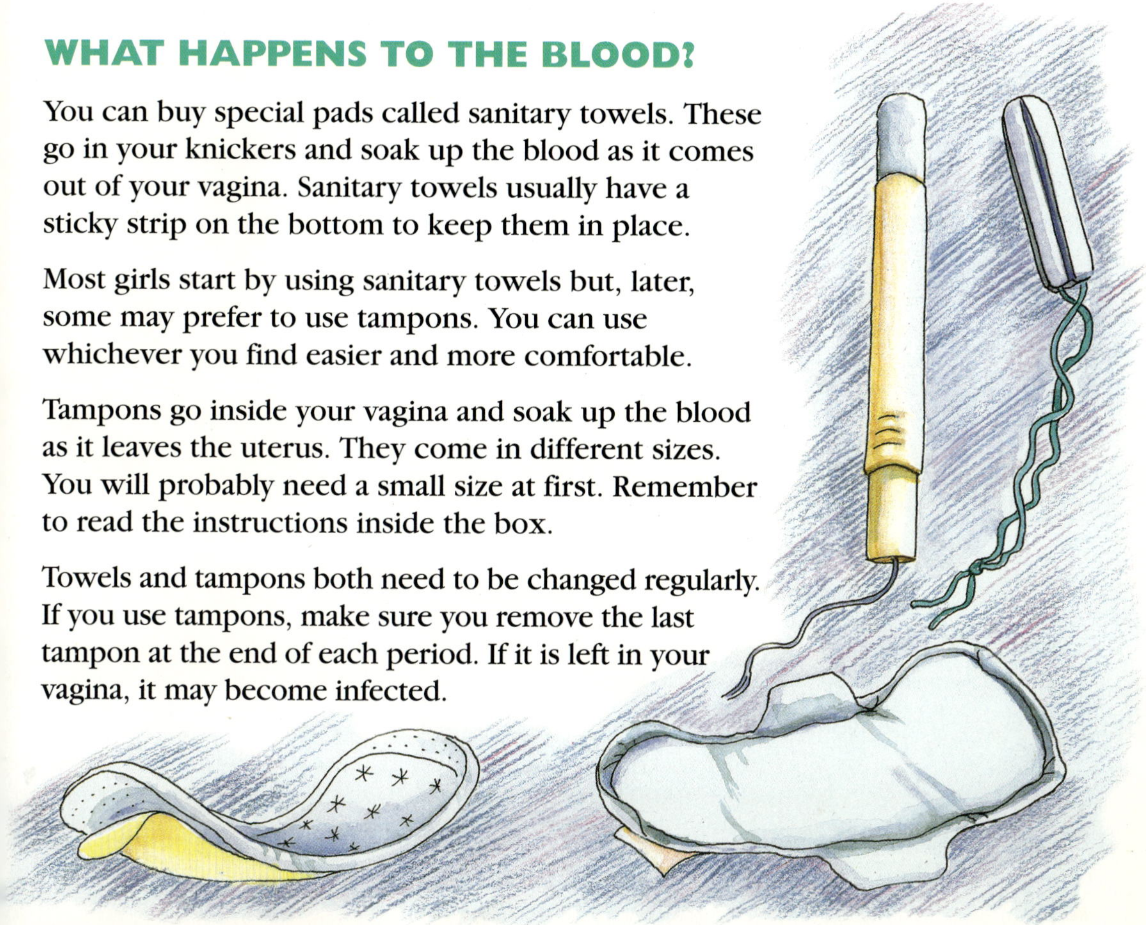

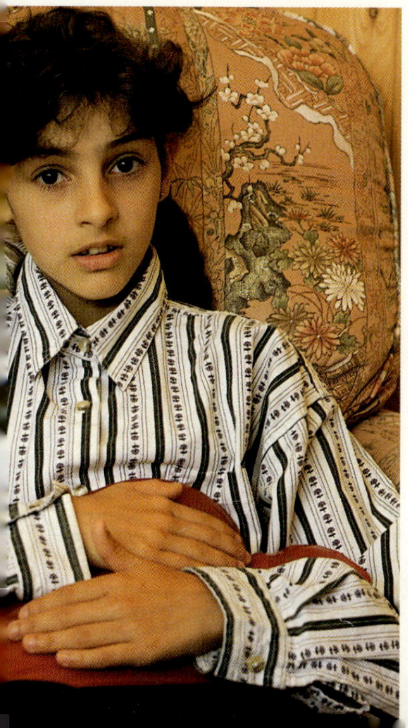

DOES IT HURT?

If you cut yourself and bleed it is painful but it is the cut that is hurting and not the blood. The blood from a period is not painful either and so, for many girls, periods do not hurt at all.

However, some girls have pains in the lower part of their tummy or backache at the start of a period. This is usually called 'period pain'.

The pain can often be helped by using a hot water bottle, taking some exercise or taking a mild painkiller such as paracetamol.

Most girls find that as they get older and start to have more regular periods they have fewer problems with period pains.

Moods and feelings

As well as having a changing body you may find that the way you feel and act changes too.

When you are a child, the way you feel and act generally stays the same. Some children are shy, some are noisy, some are happy, some are talkative. But, usually, shy children are always shy and noisy children are always noisy.

Some adolescents find that their moods seem to vary from one day to the next and this might affect the way they behave.

As you go through puberty, you might find that some days you feel really happy and want to have a good time with all your friends but other days you feel like just being on your own. Sometimes these mood changes can feel confusing.

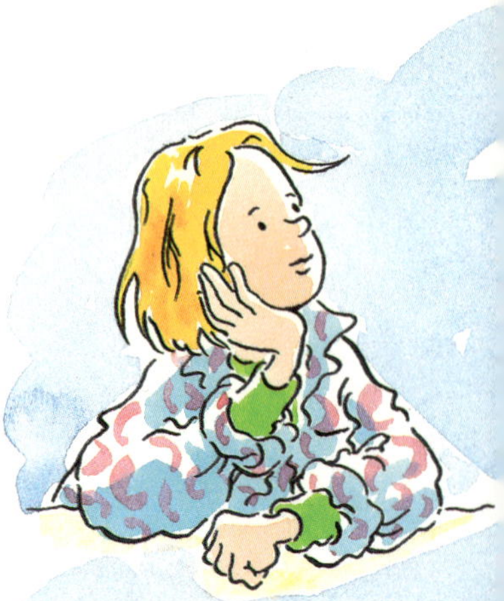

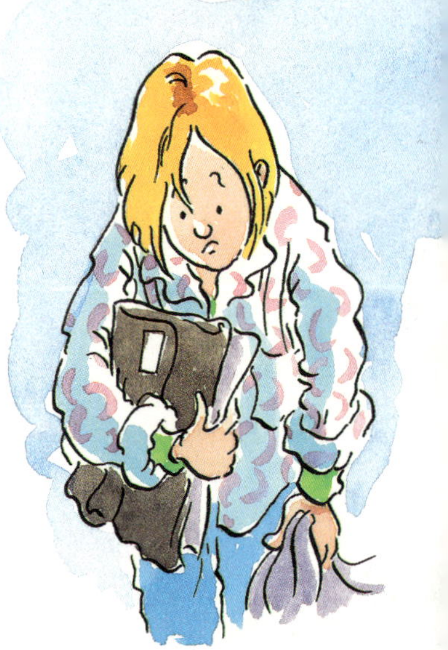

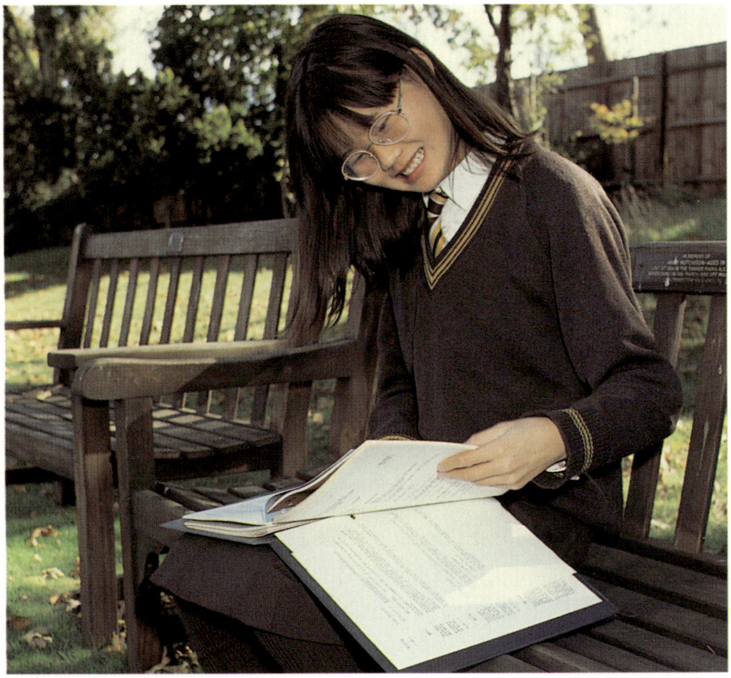

Mood changes can be confusing for people around you too. Parents may wonder why their cheerful child sometimes seems unfriendly for no real reason. Sisters can't understand why some days their brother will join in with their wild games and some days he won't.

Hormones are one of the main reasons why adolescents have mood swings.

Hormones don't just make your body change and grow. They also affect the way you feel.

You will probably find that as your hormones settle down, your moods will settle down too.

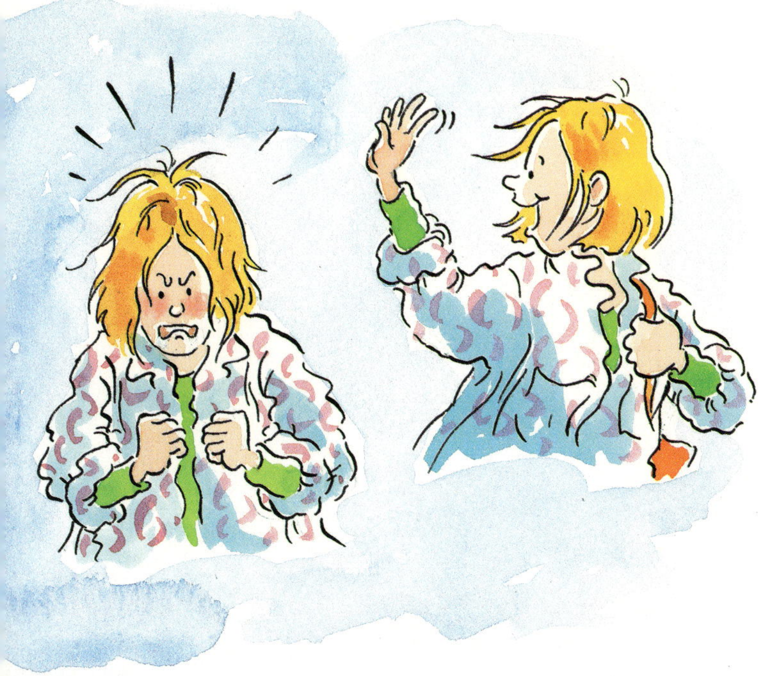

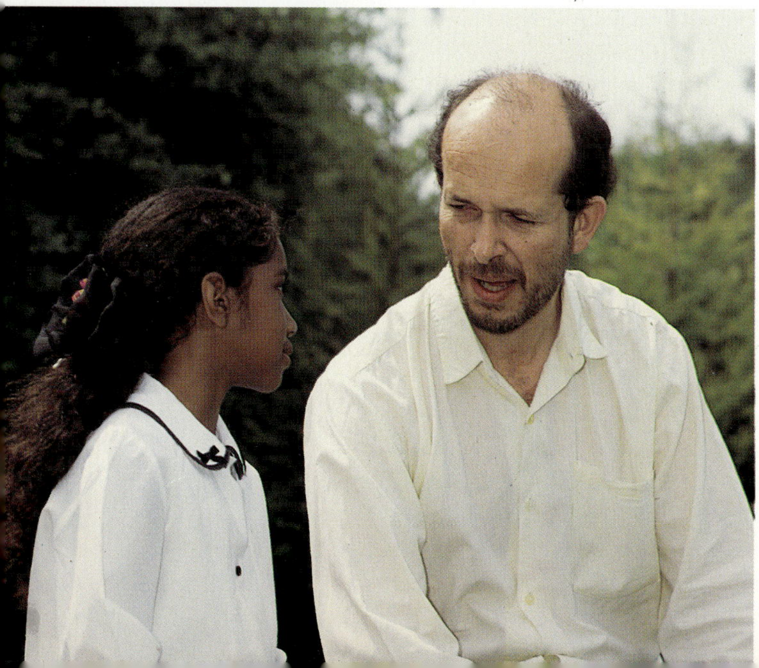

Sometimes, adolescents say that no-one understands them but people can only understand you if you share your thoughts and feelings with them.

No-one can guess how another person is feeling, especially if those feelings are changing from day to day.

COPING

One of the best ways of coping with mood changes is to talk about the way you are feeling.

Shutting yourself in your bedroom and refusing to come out is unlikely to help anyone.

Telling your parents that you really don't feel like being with everyone just at the moment and that you would prefer a bit of quiet time on your own is much more likely to help both them and you.

Talking helps them to understand how you are feeling. And most parents do want to understand.

You will probably find it helps you too. Locking your feelings away in a sort of cupboard inside you sometimes makes them seem much worse than they are.

Describing your feelings in words often unlocks that cupboard and helps you feel better about them.

Of course, this doesn't mean that you have to tell everyone everything about yourself.

Other people

As you go through puberty, you will probably start to experience much stronger feelings about other people.

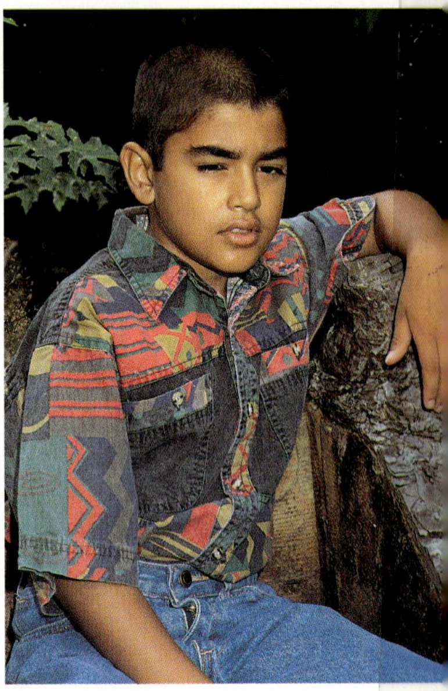

CRUSHES

Lots of adolescents begin to have crushes.

A crush is when someone becomes really special to you. You might spend a lot of time day-dreaming about this person.

A crush is not the same as having a boyfriend or girlfriend because the person you have your crush on probably doesn't feel the same way about you.

In fact, he or she may not even know you. Lots of young people have crushes on pop stars or sports personalities.

Others have crushes on people they know, like teachers or someone who lives in their street.

Girls often have crushes on other girls as well as on boys and boys have crushes on other boys as well as on girls.

Crushes are a safe, fun way to experience the strong feelings you start to have as you grow up.

You might even feel as though you are in love and you can enjoy that feeling.

But don't forget that it isn't real love.

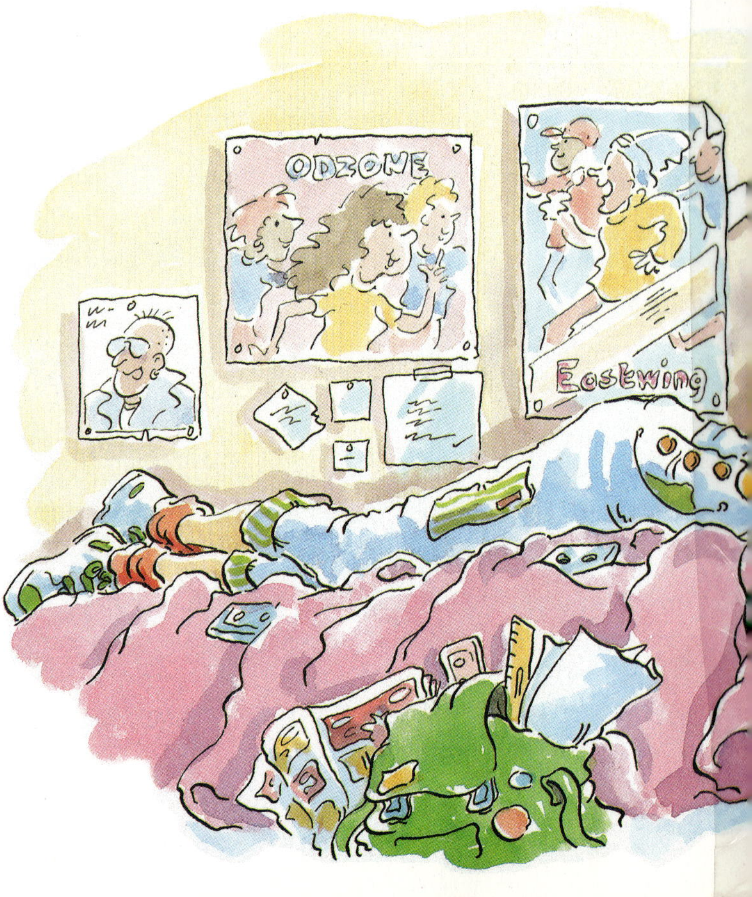

BOYFRIENDS AND GIRLFRIENDS

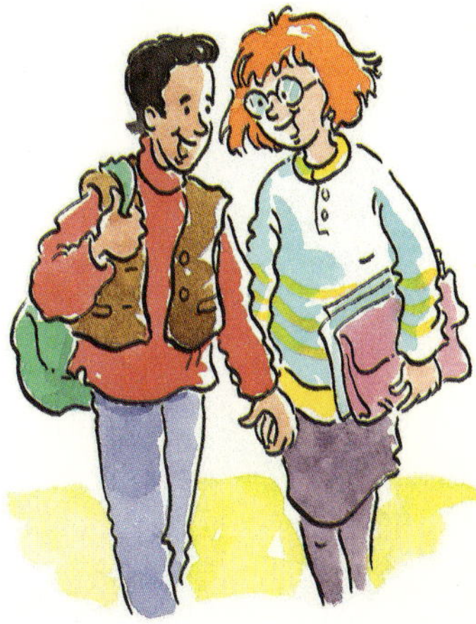

Like having a crush on someone, having a boyfriend or girlfriend means having someone who is very special to you. But this time he or she, hopefully, has the same feelings about you.

Sometimes, adolescents have the same boyfriend or girlfriend for months or even years. Others change boyfriends and girlfriends more quickly than this.

There is no rule that says you have to have a boyfriend or girlfriend. Lots of perfectly normal adolescents don't have one.

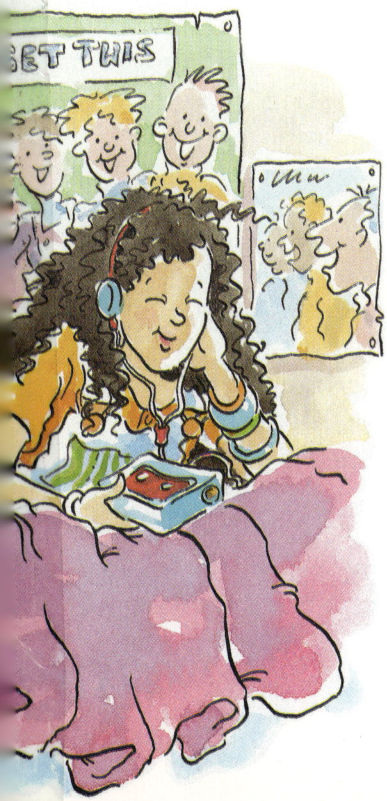

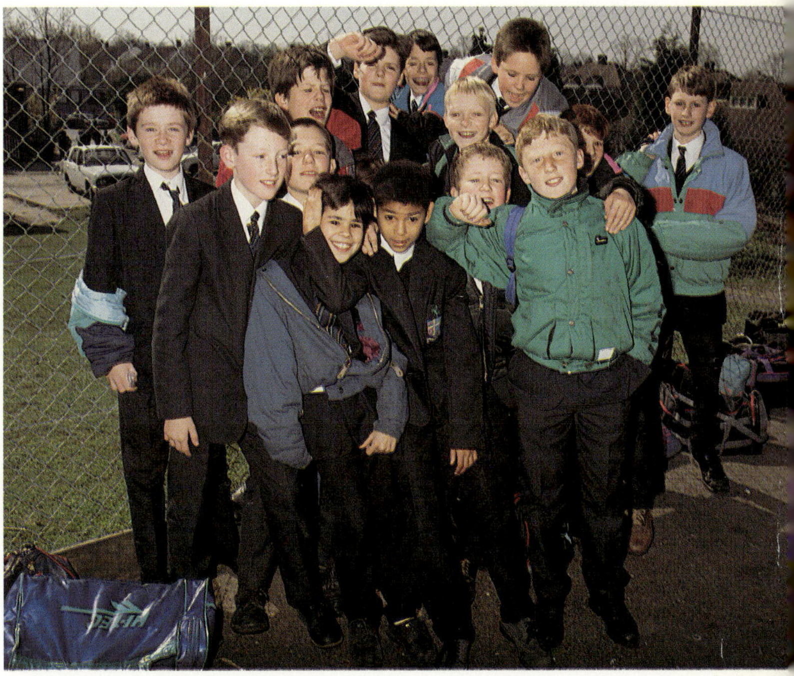

Some children worry because they don't have a boyfriend or girlfriend or perhaps because they don't have many friends at all.

They wonder whether changing the way they look or act might make them more popular.

But the best way to get on with people is just to be yourself. Like yourself and others will like you too.

Sex

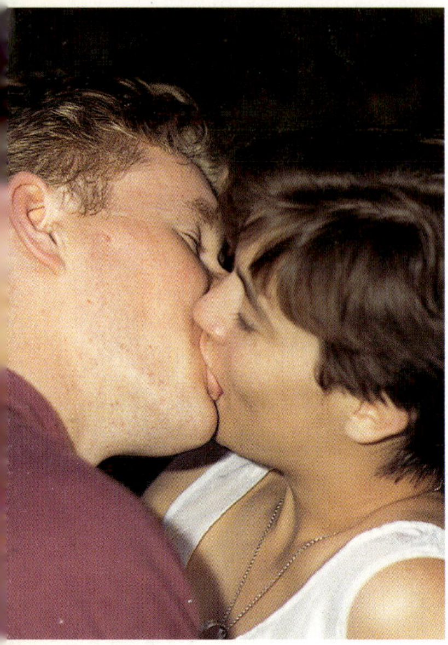

When you are older, you may find that someone becomes particularly special to you. Your feelings about that person will probably become stronger and stronger.

Lots of people call this feeling 'being in love'.

Two people who are in love will often think of themselves as a couple, as two people who love and respect each other.

As their love grows stronger, they may eventually decide that they want to do more than kiss and cuddle.

This may mean that that they would like, and are ready, to have sexual intercourse.

Sexual intercourse is known by lots of different names:

- Often it is just shortened to the word 'sex'.
- Some people call it 'making love' because it is a way of feeling very close to someone you love.
- Others call it 'sleeping together' because it usually happens in bed.

WHAT HAPPENS DURING SEX?

Kissing and cuddling can give a man an erection. It can also make a woman's vagina produce more vaginal fluid.

When this happens, the man and woman may decide that they would like to make love.

One way to do this is for the woman to lie on her back with the man on top. The man faces her and slides his penis into her vagina. Either the man, the woman or both of them move their hips to make the penis slip up and down in the vagina.

Eventually the man is likely to ejaculate and his semen will squirt out into the woman's vagina.

At the same time he will probably have a feeling called an orgasm. The woman may have an orgasm too.

An orgasm is like an excited feeling that builds up and up inside a person. It reaches a peak and then goes away, leaving the person feeling very relaxed.

BEING IN CHARGE

Deciding to have sex with someone is a very important decision to make.

It is something that both people should talk about first and not something that 'just happens'.

Either person or both people can decide that they don't want to have sex. Nobody has to have sex. It's your body. You decide what to do with it.

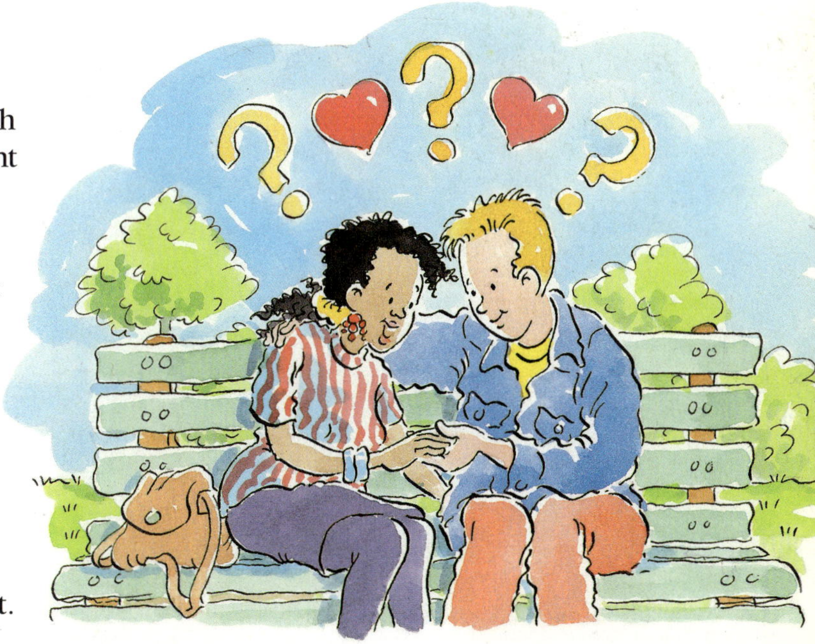

Most countries have a law that tells you the youngest age at which people are allowed to have sex. In Great Britain it is 16.

This does not mean that people have to have sex when they are 16.

Many religions also have rules about sex, such as not having sex until you are married.

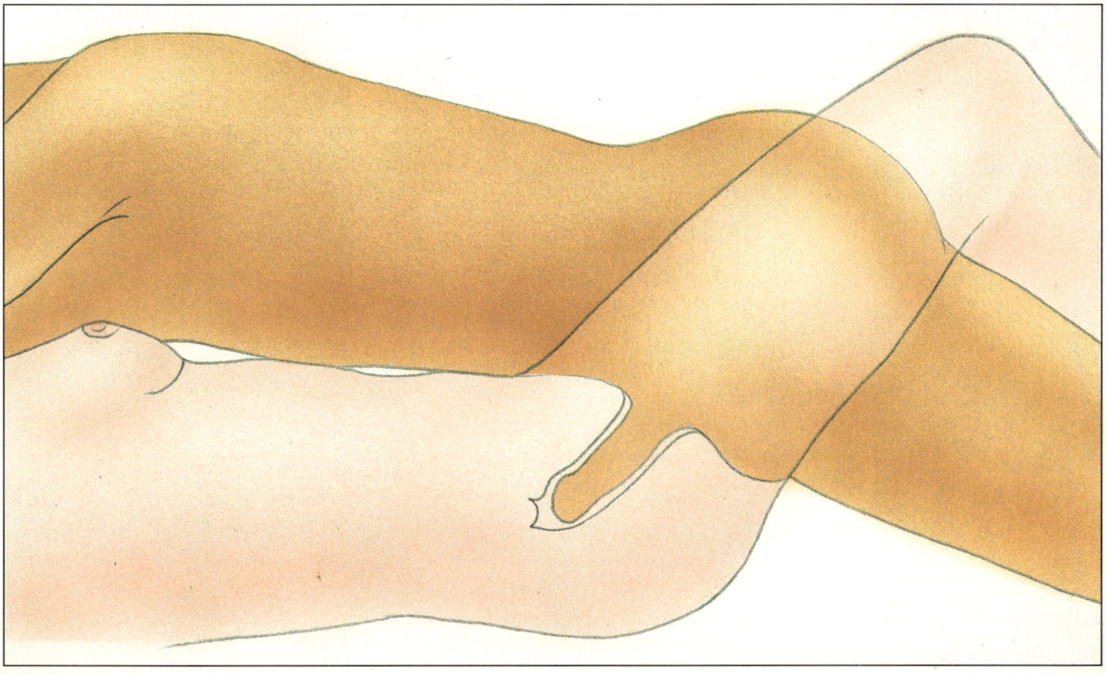

More about sex

WHY DO PEOPLE HAVE SEX?

The main reason why our bodies change and grow is so that men and women can, between them, make a baby.

Having sex is the beginning of having a baby.

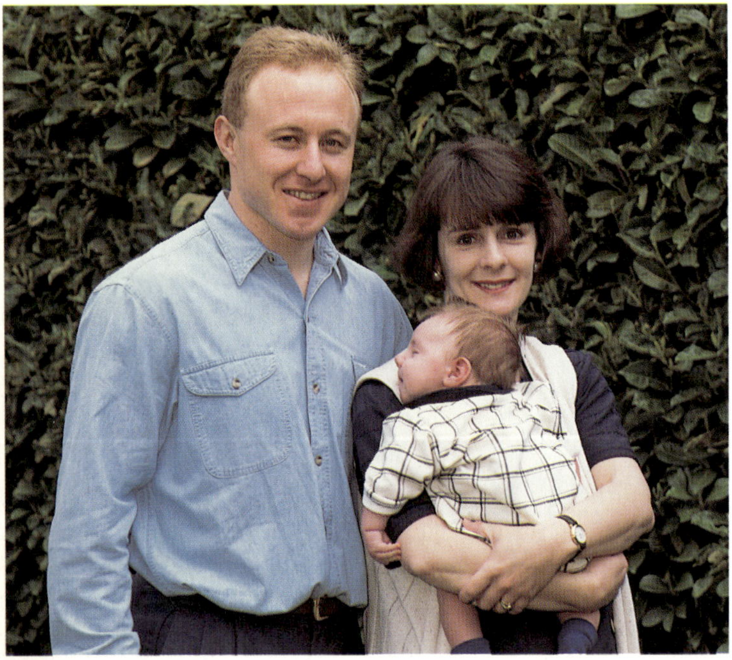

HOW DOES A NEW BABY START?

During sexual intercourse, if one of the sperm in the man's semen meets and joins up with one of the woman's eggs they may settle down and grow in the woman's uterus. This is the start of a baby.

Having sex also feels good too.

Not everyone who has sex wants, or is ready for, a baby. People who want to have sex but don't want to have a baby can use something called contraception.

Before two people have sex they need to know about contraception and also about protecting themselves against certain infections.

WHAT IS CONTRACEPTION?

Lots of couples decide that although they would like to make love together they are not ready to have a baby. So, to prevent a baby being made they either have to stop the sperm and the egg coming together or stop the sperm and egg settling down in the uterus.

There are lots of ways of doing this and they are known as methods of contraception. The main methods are described on pages 28 and 29.

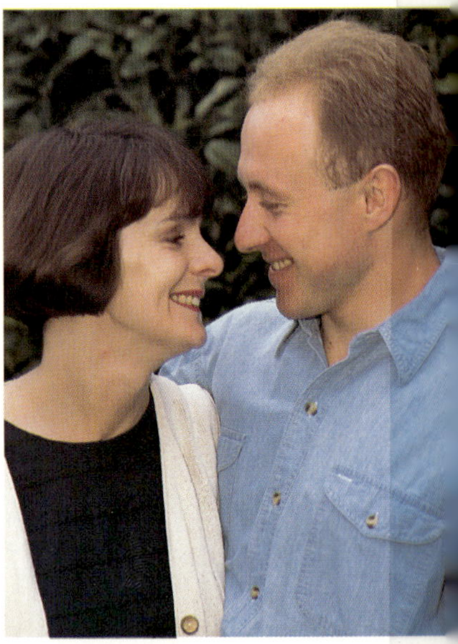

SEXUALLY TRANSMITTED DISEASES

Sometimes germs or infections get into semen or vaginal fluids. These infections can pass from one person to another during sex. Because of this they are often called sexually transmitted diseases.

Although doctors can cure most sexually transmitted diseases using medicines, it is better to try not to get them in the first place.

The best way to do this is to use a condom, which stops infected semen or vaginal fluid from getting into another person's body.

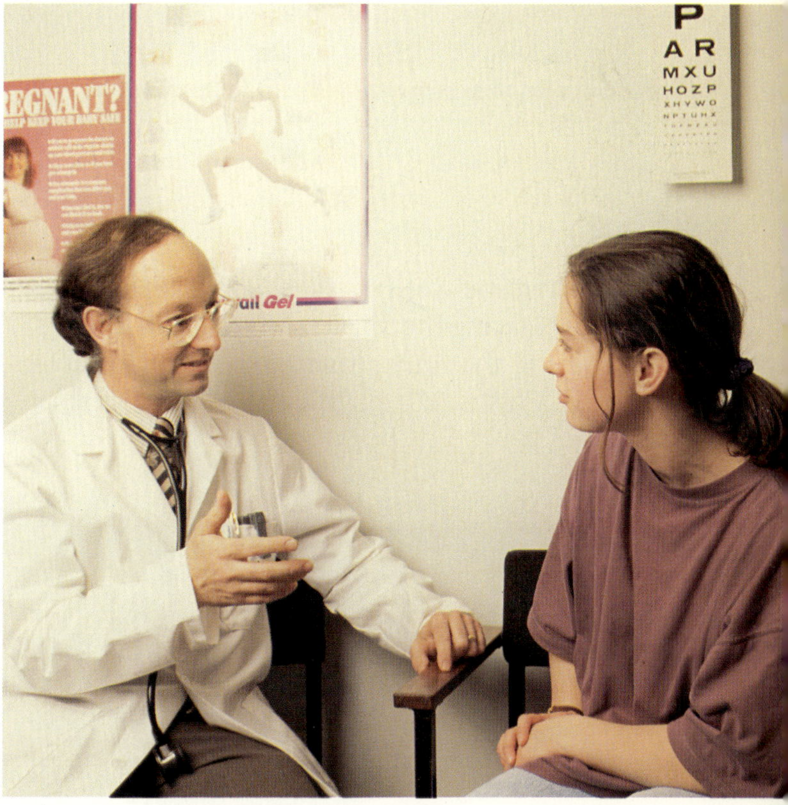

You can find out more about condoms on the next page.

ANY QUESTIONS?

If a man has an erection does he have to have sex?
No. An erection will usually go away after a short while.

Does sex hurt the woman?
Not usually. The vagina is very stretchy and the extra fluid it has produced makes it slippery so that the penis can slide in.

Can urine come out of a man's penis at the same time as semen?
No. A special muscle at the bottom of the penis stops this happening.

If you have any other questions, you could talk to your parents or a teacher.

Contraception

Stopping a baby from being made is called contraception. A couple who do not want a baby should use some form of contraception when they make love. This page and the next describe the main types of contraception.

Sometimes young people hear all sorts of stories about other ways to stop a baby being made. Most of them are not true.

Doctors and family planning clinics are there to talk to people about contraception. Parents can give advice too.

THE PILL

This is a pill that the woman takes. Some types of pill stop any eggs leaving the woman's ovaries. Some make changes to the fluid around the cervix, or neck of the uterus. This makes it difficult for any sperm to get through.

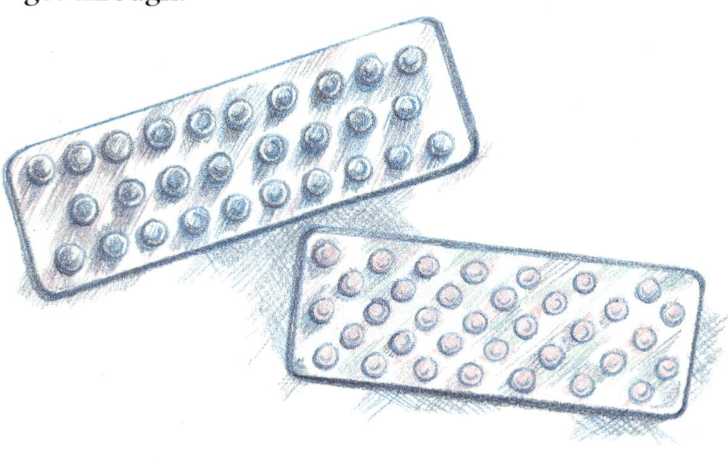

All types make changes in the uterus lining so that if a sperm and egg did meet they wouldn't be able to settle down there.

In order for the pill to work the woman has to remember to take it. Some types are taken every day. Some are taken for three weeks with one week off.

Injections and implants, which don't have to be taken every day but last for a long time, are available too. These work in the same way as the pill.

THE CONDOM

A man's condom looks a bit like a long balloon that hasn't been blown up.

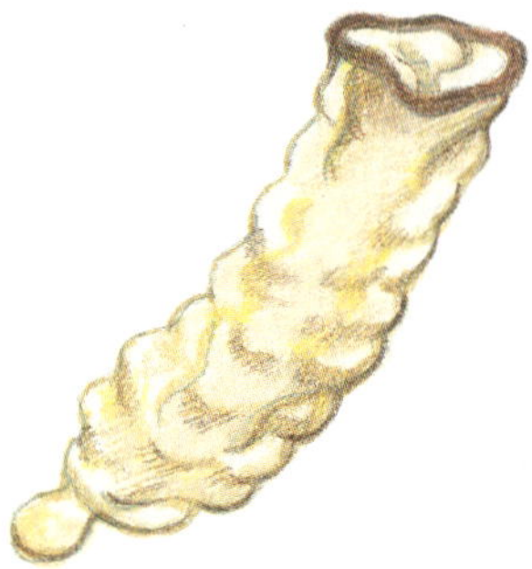

When a man has an erection the condom is rolled down over his penis before the couple make love. Then, when he ejaculates, all the semen is caught inside the condom and the sperm can't reach the egg.

There is a condom for women too. This fits inside her vagina and, like the man's condom, catches all the semen.

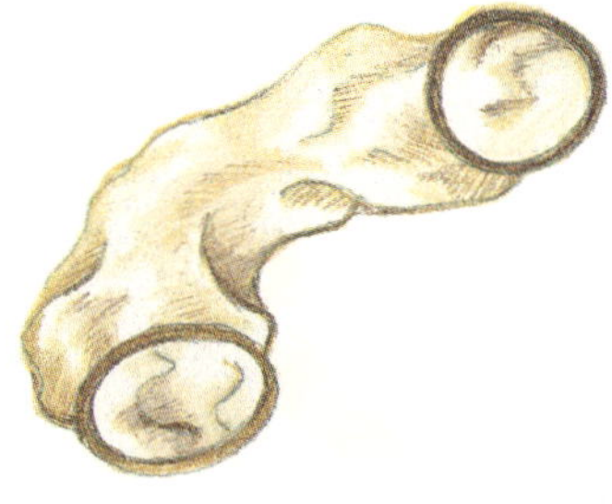

A new condom has to be used each time a couple make love.

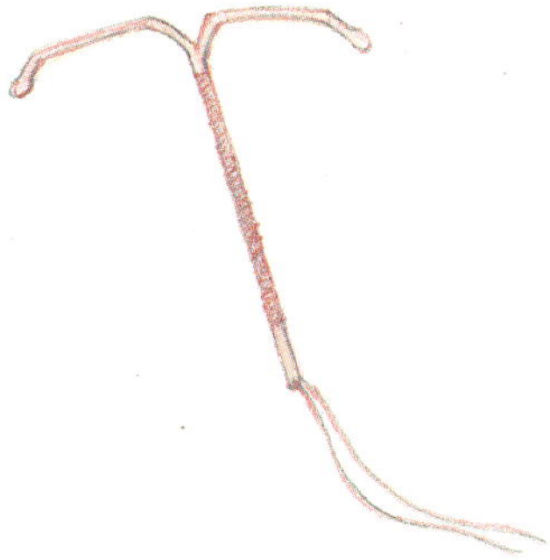

THE IUD

IUD stands for Intra-Uterine Device. An IUD is very small and put inside the uterus by a doctor.

It is usually made of narrow pieces of plastic with thin copper wire wrapped around them. The copper in the IUD probably stops the sperm and egg joining together. If any did meet, the IUD would stop them settling in the uterus. The same IUD can stay in the uterus for a number of years.

THE CAP OR DIAPHRAGM

This small rubber dome fits over the woman's cervix.

It has to be put in before a couple make love and stops any semen from getting into her uterus.

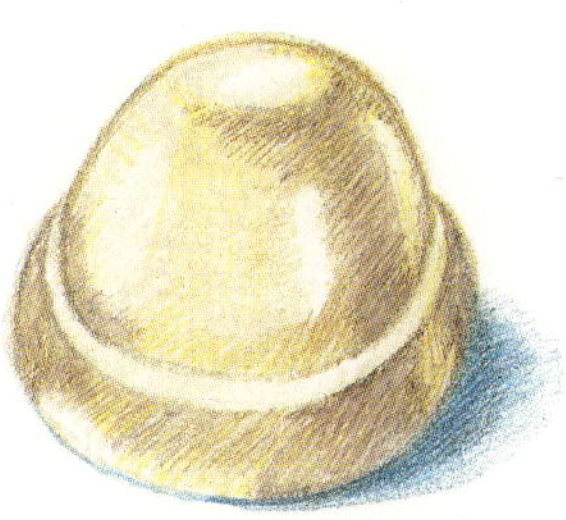

This means that the sperm can't swim up to the egg.

It has to be used every time a couple make love.

THE 'EMERGENCY' PILL

If a couple make love without contraception or if something goes wrong with the contraception they have used, such as the condom tearing, they should go and see a doctor.

If they go within three days, the woman can be given pills that work in the same way as the ordinary pill.

It is not meant to be used as a couple's main form of contraception and it makes some women feel rather sick. It is only meant to be used in an emergency.

NATURAL METHODS

Some people may feel that the types of contraception mentioned so far are not natural and are wrong.

A baby can only be made if a sperm meets an egg in the fallopian tube.

There are only about five days every month when this could happen.

If a couple don't make love during these five days, then the woman probably won't get pregnant.

Some people use this as a type of contraception. It is sometimes called the rhythm method or natural contraception.

The problem is that it is very difficult to know when these five days are and so it is not a reliable way of stopping a woman from becoming pregnant.

A new life

Of course, there are times when a couple do want to have a baby. Then they have sex without using contraception.

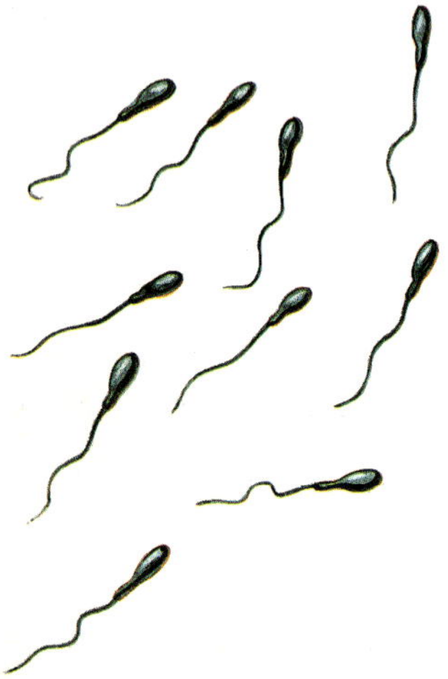

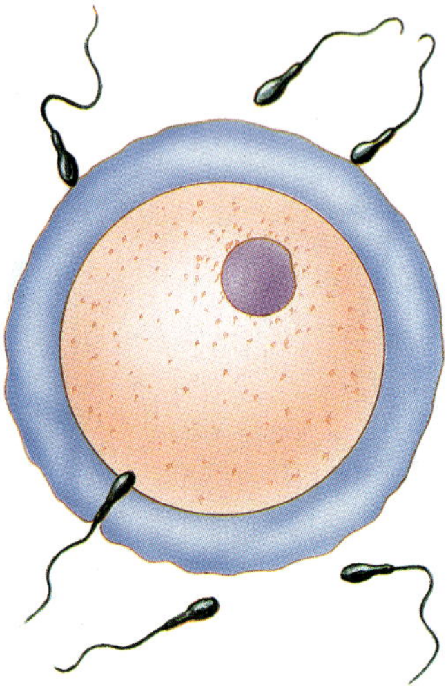

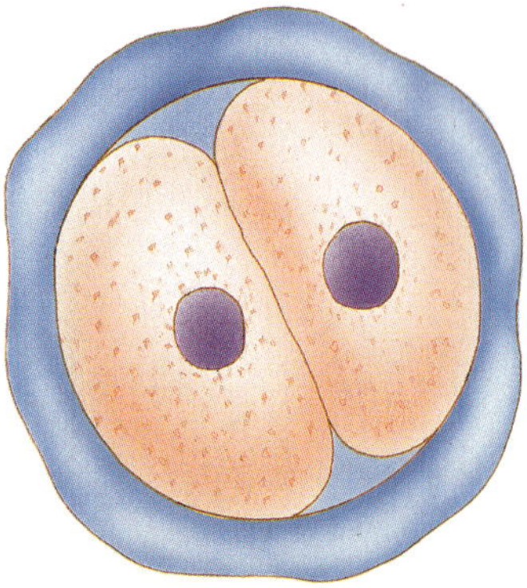

When a couple make love and the man ejaculates, the sperm that are in his semen start swimming up through the woman's uterus.

Their job is to find and reach an egg in the woman's fallopian tube. If there is one, the first sperm to get to the egg wriggles inside. This sperm and the egg join together to form a new cell.

This cell divides into two. The two cells split to make four cells. The cells keep on splitting until there is a little ball of cells.

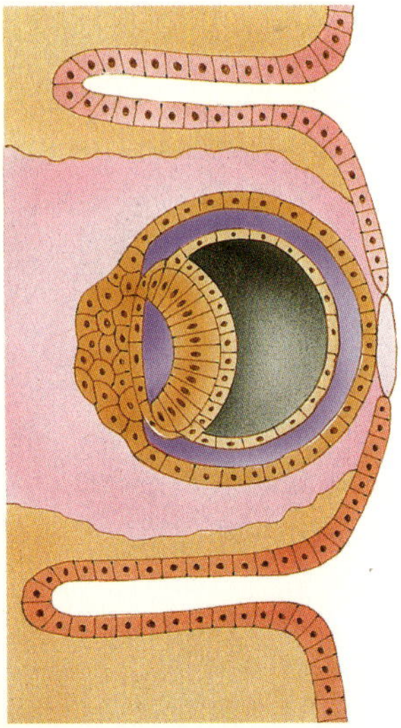

The ball of cells travels down the fallopian tube and into the uterus. There, it settles down in the soft lining which has been thickened with extra blood vessels.

Once this happens, the woman is said to be pregnant.

The ball of cells then continues to grow and develop until it becomes a baby.

Once the ball of cells has settled down in the uterus, the woman's body knows not to shed the lining of her uterus. So, often, the first thing a woman notices when she is pregnant is that she does not have her period.

Her body also knows to stop releasing any more eggs. A woman has no periods when she is pregnant.

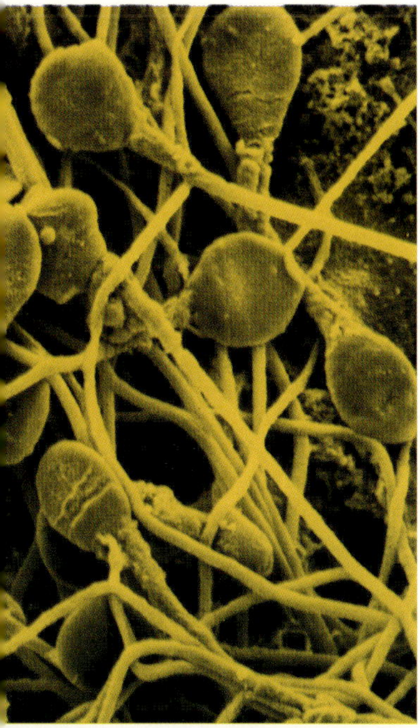

Sperm showing head and tail sections

There are special tests called pregnancy tests that can tell whether or not a woman is going to have a baby.

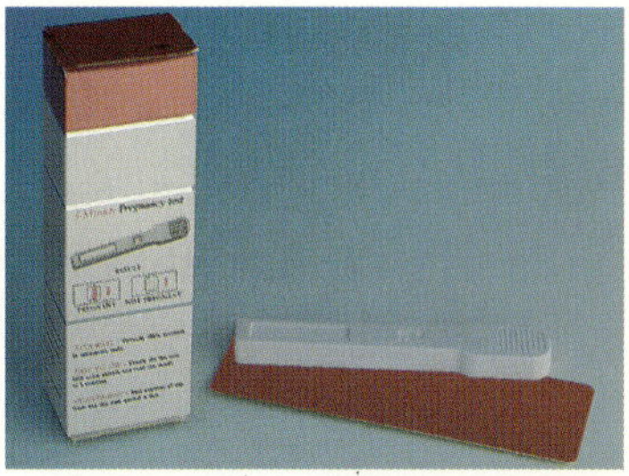

A pregnancy testing kit can be bought at a chemist. A doctor or nurse could do the test as well.

When you are pregnant there are changes in your urine. The tests check to see whether these changes have happened.

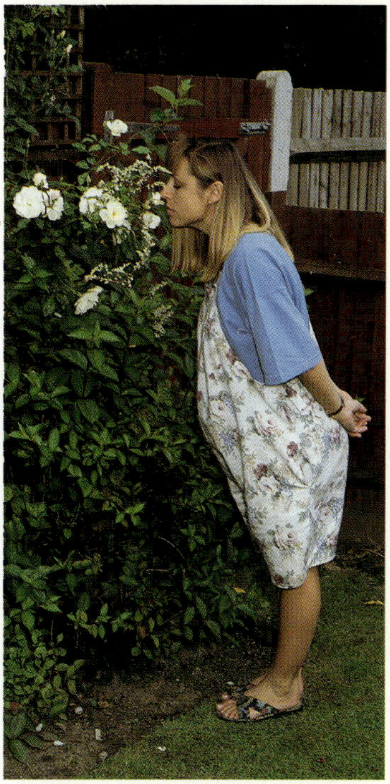

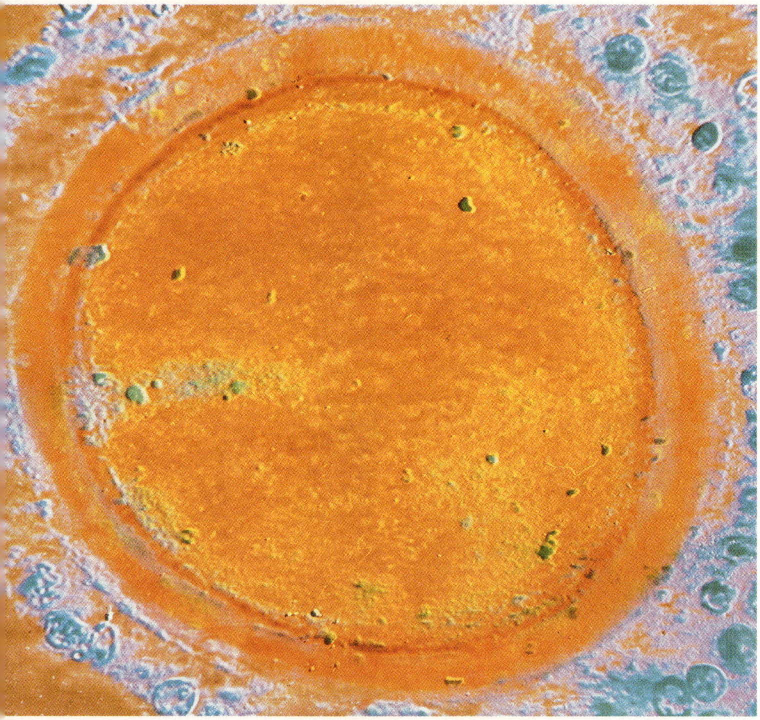

Human egg surrounded by sperm

Some women feel very sick when they are first pregnant.

This usually happens in the morning but it can happen at other times of the day.

This feeling usually wears off during pregnancy.

Pregnancy

The little ball of cells that has settled down in the wall of the uterus continues to grow.

The uterus will be its home for the next nine months (around 40 weeks) as it develops into a baby.

For about the first eight weeks it is called an embryo.

At four weeks the embryo looks a bit like a tadpole. It is about 2mm long.

Where the ball of cells settled in the lining of the uterus, a special pocket filled with blood is starting to grow. This is the placenta.

The embryo is attached to the placenta by a cord. This is called the umbilical cord. Blood passes between a mother and her baby through the placenta and along the umbilical cord bringing food and oxygen to the baby.

At eight weeks the embryo looks much more like a baby, although it is still only about the size of a grown-up's thumbnail.

The embryo is floating in a bag of liquid. This bag is known as the amniotic sac. It helps to protect the embryo from any knocks and bumps.

Babies growing in the uterus do not need to breathe air in the same way that we do. They get their oxygen from their mother's blood.

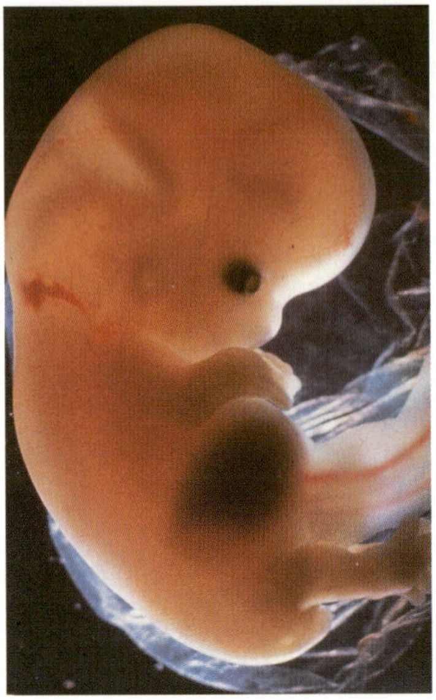

Embryo at about seven weeks

At twenty weeks the baby is about the same length as a new pencil but much bendier!

It has fingers and toes and has started to grow hair, eyelashes and eyebrows.

By now the mother has probably felt the baby kicking inside her.

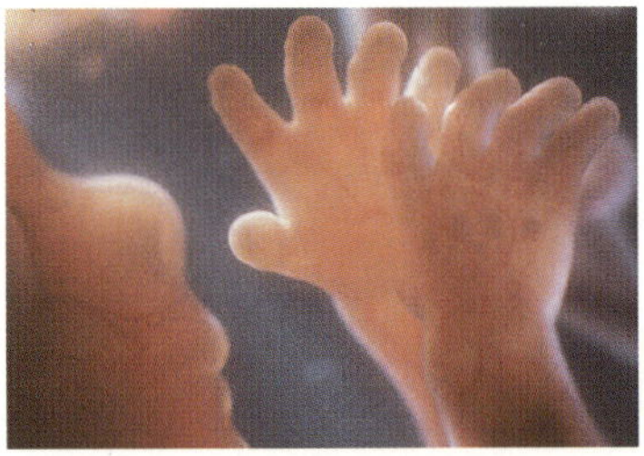

At twenty weeks the baby's fingers have begun to develop.

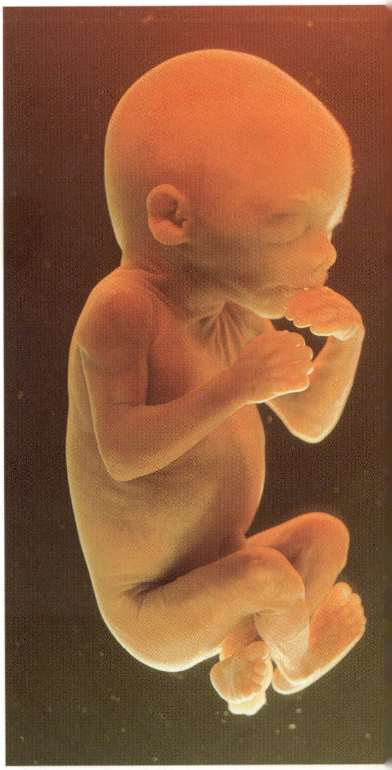

Baby at about twenty weeks.

By about thirty-two weeks the baby is starting to get itself into position to be born.

The mother's uterus has had to stretch quite a lot. Most women have quite a large bulge in front of them by this stage.

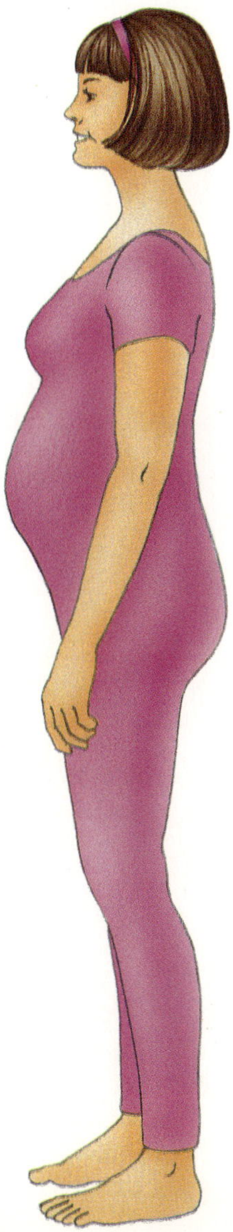

At about forty weeks the baby is ready to be born.

Muscles in the woman's uterus start to work. These open up her cervix so that the baby's head can come through and they start to push the baby downwards.

The baby pushes through the cervix, then down through her vagina and out through her vaginal opening.

This all takes several hours.

After the baby has been born, the placenta comes away from the lining of the uterus and comes out through the woman's vagina.

When the baby is born it is still attached to the mother by its umbilical cord. The cord is then cut. It doesn't hurt the baby or mother at all.

The place where the umbilical cord started eventually becomes the baby's tummy button, or navel.

Having a baby is very hard work for both the mother and the baby. The hard work doesn't stop there. Young babies demand a lot of attention and are a big responsibility. Life for the baby's parents will never be the same again!

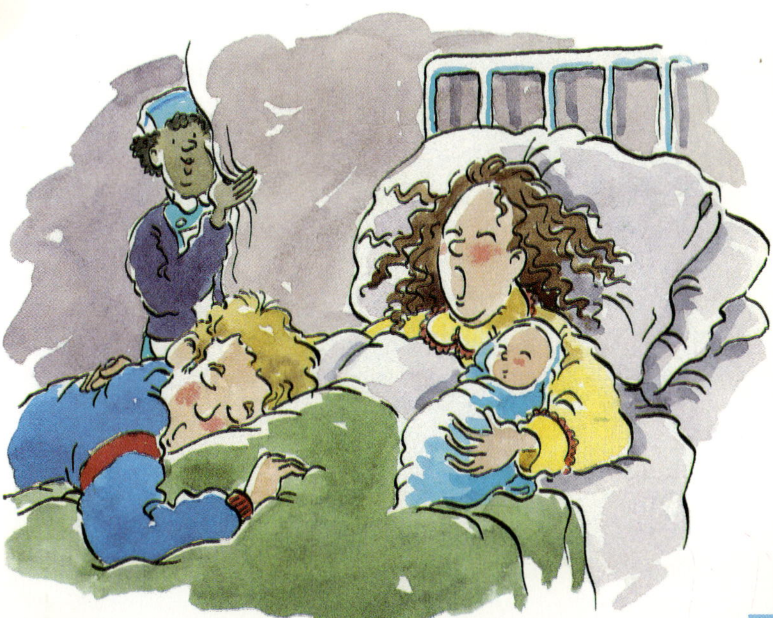

HIV and AIDS

You will probably have heard of the word AIDS and the initials HIV but, like many people, you may not be sure exactly what they are or what they mean.

The word AIDS comes from the phrase Acquired Immuno-Deficiency Syndrome. The first letters of these words have been put together to make a new word.

This is what Acquired Immuno-Deficiency Syndrome means.

A **Acquired means something a person has got from someone else.**

I **Immuno means that it has something to do with the immune system. The immune system is the body's way of protecting itself from illness.**

D **Deficiency means that something is not working properly.**

S **Syndrome means a collection of signs or symptoms of illness.**

So, Acquired Immuno-Deficiency Syndrome means signs that something has got into the body that is stopping the immune system from working properly.

That something is a virus called HIV or Human Immuno-deficiency Virus. A virus is like a germ or bug that gets into the body.

Sometimes people with HIV start to get very ill. They may go on to develop AIDS.

Doctors have come up with a list of illnesses that mean that a person has AIDS. Many of the people who have AIDS will die.

Most people with HIV are, however, perfectly fit and healthy.

Having HIV is not the same thing as having AIDS.

But HIV is a very serious virus. It can lead to death and at the moment it cannot be cured.

Doctors are hoping to find a medicine that will do this or a vaccine that will protect people from HIV.

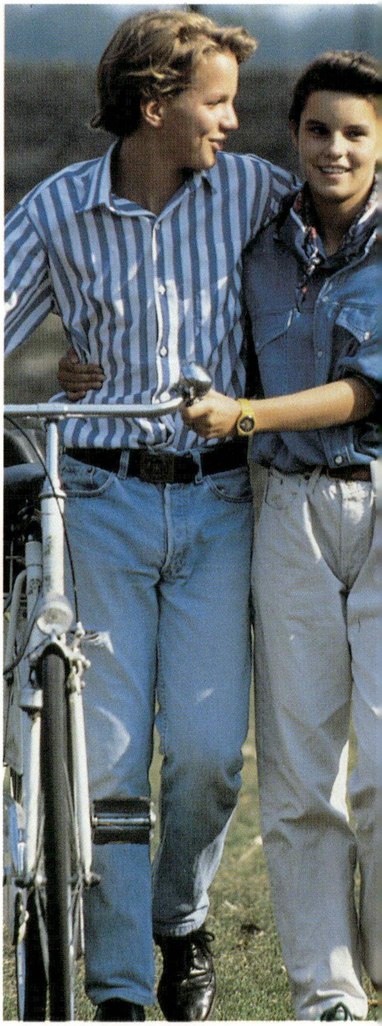

You cannot tell whether someone has HIV just by looking at them.

HOW PEOPLE GET HIV

There are only a few ways that the HIV virus is passed from one person to another.

By understanding how to protect themselves, most people can avoid any risk of getting the virus.

HIV lives in blood, semen and vaginal fluids.

In blood

You can only get HIV from blood if the blood of a person with the virus gets into your bloodstream, for example, through a cut or a graze. It is a sensible idea to get an adult to deal with any accident that involves blood. Adults should take care to deal with blood carefully.

The needles in injections go into the bloodstream but doctors, dentists and nurses always use needles just once and then they throw them away.

Needles that have been used for one person should ***never*** be used for someone else.

Never touch a needle or syringe that you see lying about. Tell an adult about it and ask them to throw it away properly.

In semen and vaginal fluids

HIV can be passed between two people when they have sex. They best way to stop this happening is to use a condom.

A condom stops any semen from getting into the other person's body. It also stops any vaginal fluids from getting onto the penis.

Babies

Babies whose mothers have HIV can be born with the virus. HIV can also be passed on to the baby through its mother's breastmilk.

HOW PEOPLE DON'T GET HIV

You *cannot* get HIV from touching, shaking hands, hugging or kissing a person with HIV.

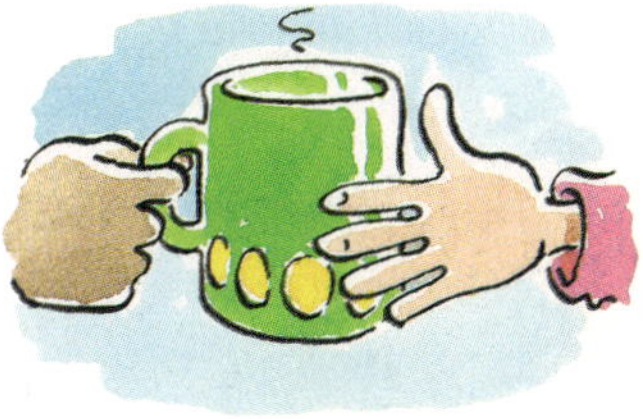

You *cannot* get HIV from sharing cups, knives and forks, food or towels with a person with HIV.

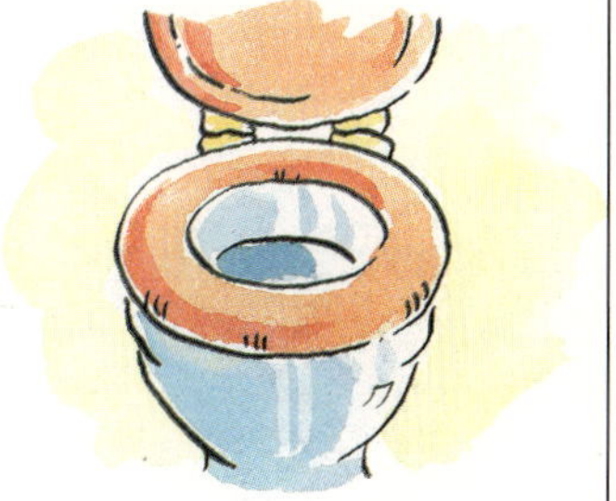

You *cannot* get HIV from swimming pools or toilet seats.

You *cannot* get HIV from someone coughing or sneezing on you.

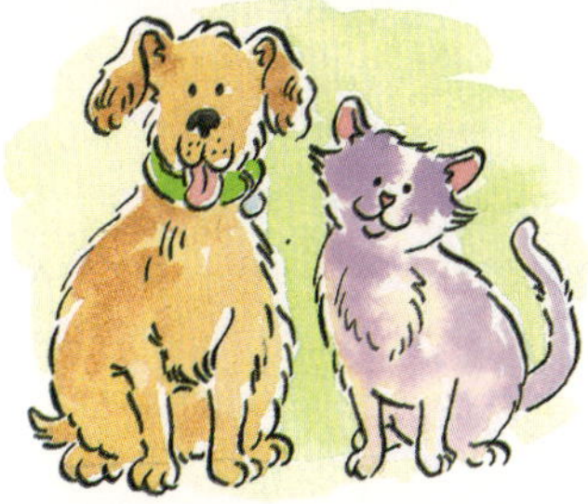

You *cannot* get HIV from insect bites, dogs, cats or other domestic animals.

Friends

Adolescence is a time when friends and friendships become very important.

Most children enjoy having friends but the centre of their life is usually their family.

The things they like doing are probably the things that the other members of their family enjoy too.

The food they eat, the clothes they wear and the way they speak are all likely to be influenced by the way their particular family lives its life.

Part of growing up is about learning to be an individual. Not just someone's son or daughter or someone's brother or sister, but you.

At the start of this process, many children find that instead of having a feeling of belonging only to their family they also get a feeling of belonging with other people of their own age.

Now it's not just your family who influence you but your friends too.

Lots of adolescents like to wear the same sort of clothes, listen to the same sort of music and act in the same way as their friends.

This is fine. It makes you feel part of a group and being part of a group makes you feel liked and wanted.

But don't think you always have to go along with everyone else if you don't want to.

If you don't feel right in green and purple trainers, you don't have to wear them.

If you don't like the music that everyone else thinks is brilliant, then you don't have to pretend you do.

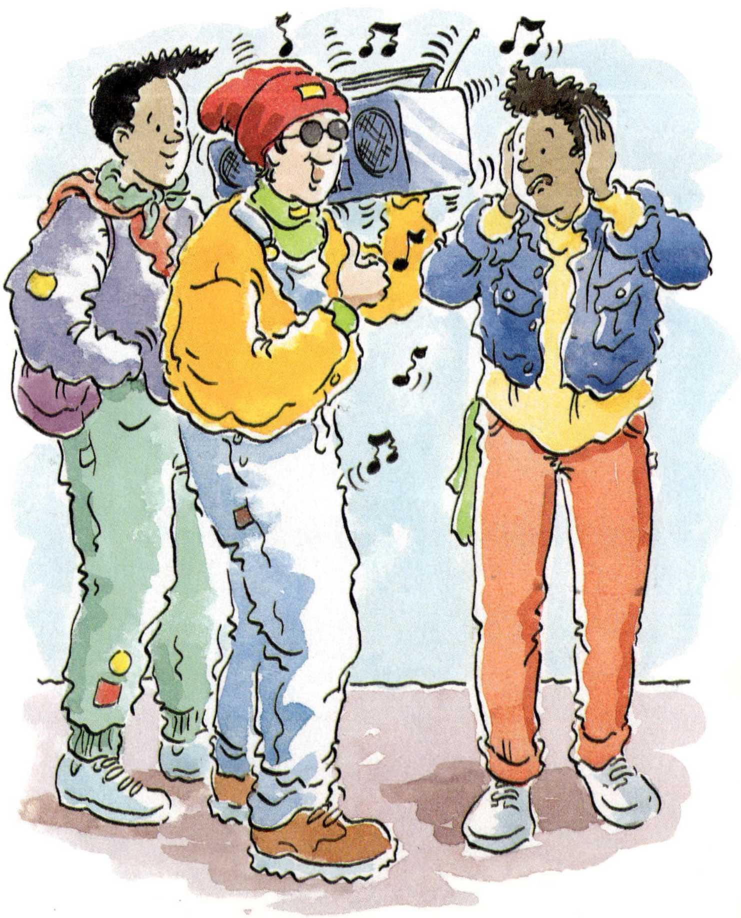

MAKING YOUR OWN MIND UP

Sometimes people do things that they know they shouldn't or things they would really rather not do just because they don't want to be different.

But behaving like this doesn't usually make you feel very good. It often just makes you feel guilty and cross with yourself for being weak.

Sometimes these situations arise when one person asks another to do something that is wrong or bad for you, such as stealing, smoking or drinking.

You'll find some information about smoking, alcohol and drugs on the next few pages of this book.

It is often much easier to say no to something if you can give good reasons explaining why you don't want to do it.

And if people say they won't be your friends if you don't do something then they are not true friends.

Knowing when to go along with everyone else and when to make up your own mind about things is an important skill to learn.

FRIENDS FOR EVER?

Some people find that adolescence is a time when they make strong and lasting friendships. Others find that it is a time when friendships come and go.

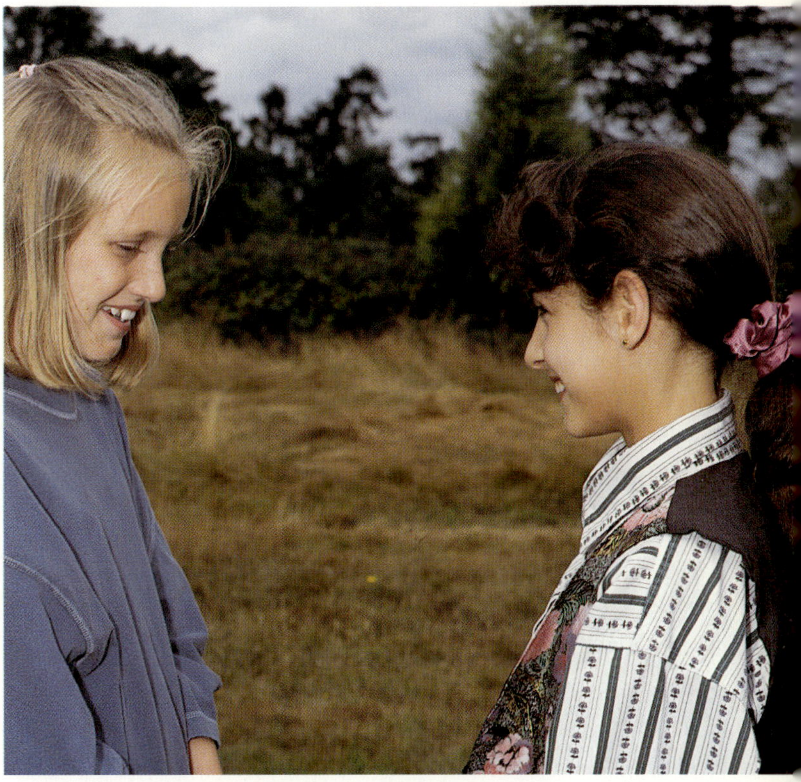

As you go through adolescence, you will probably find that your interests and way of behaving are changing. This will be happening to your friends too and sometimes you simply grow apart.

But, just as two people can grow apart, so two people can grow together and new friendships are formed.

Smoking

Every year, in Britain, over 100,000 people die early from diseases that they probably got from smoking.

That's more than 2,000 people a week or about 300 every day.

The diseases you can get from smoking include lung cancer, bronchitis and heart attacks.

The smoke from cigarettes is made up of three main ingredients: nicotine, carbon monoxide and tar.

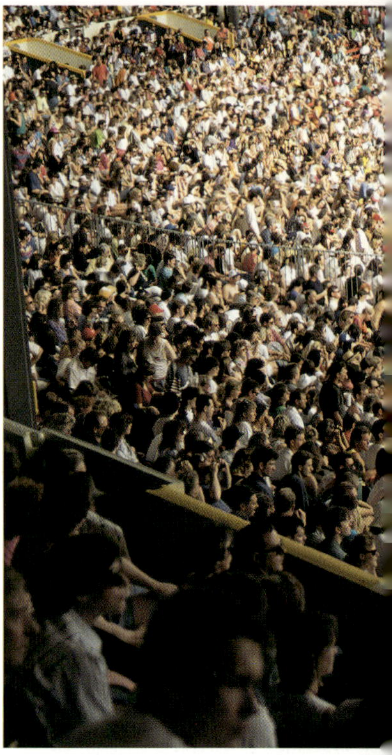

NICOTINE When someone breathes in cigarette smoke, the nicotine goes straight into the bloodstream.

Nicotine can make the heart beat faster than it should. It can also make it more difficult for the heart to push the blood around the bloodstream. This makes the heart work too hard and wears it out.

Nicotine can be addictive. This means that, although the nicotine is harming it, the person's body starts to need the nicotine.

CARBON MONOXIDE Carbon monoxide is what comes out of the end of a car's exhaust. It is a poisonous gas.

Healthy blood has lots of oxygen in it. Some of the oxygen in a smoker's blood is replaced by carbon monoxide. This makes the blood less able to keep the body in good condition.

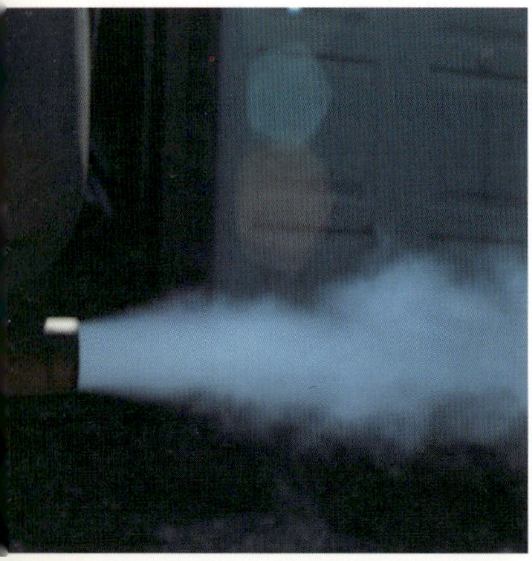

Carbon monoxide is also thought to lead to a smoker's blood vessels becoming blocked. This can cause heart problems and mean that the blood does not flow around the bloodstream properly.

TAR Tar is a black, sticky liquid. It is often used in road laying. Although you can't see any black tar in cigarette smoke, when the smoke gets to the lungs the tiny specks join together to form a black coating.

Tar can cause cancer. It can also cause terrible damage to the lungs and affect a smoker's breathing.

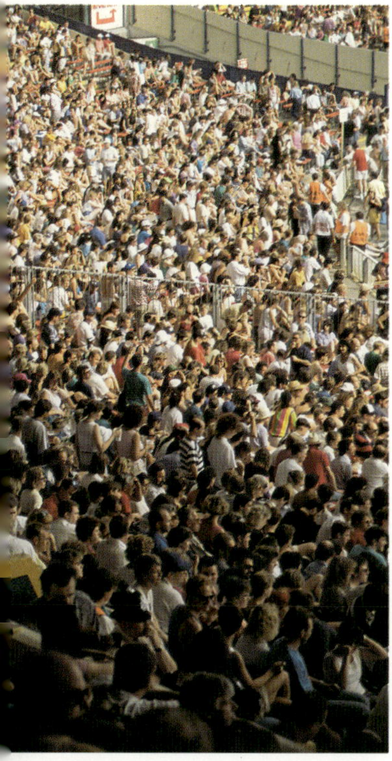

MORE REASONS TO SAY NO

People sometimes start smoking because they think it makes them look grown up and cool.

But it is far more grown up to make a decision not to smoke because you know how much it can harm your body and to stick to that decision.

As for looking cool, there are better ways of looking cool than dangling some burning, dried leaves between your fingers.

Smoking is expensive and smelly too. It makes your hair smell, your clothes smell and your breath smell.

Being smelly is definitely not cool.

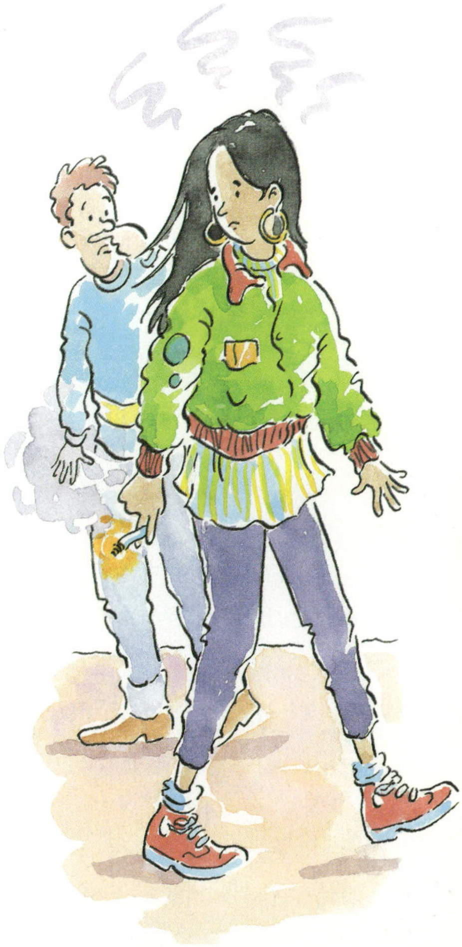

PASSIVE SMOKING

When people smoke, only some of the smoke goes into their own lungs. The rest goes into the air.

Breathing in smoky air is sometimes called passive smoking.

Passive smoking may make people cough or sneeze, feel dizzy or give them a headache.

It may lead to more serious health problems.

Many people are worried about passive smoking. Smoking is being banned in more and more places, such as on buses and trains, so that people don't have to breathe in smoky air.

If around 300 people a day die an early death from diseases that are linked to smoking, someone else will probably have lost his or her life while you were reading this page.

Alcohol

Drinks can be put into two groups: alcoholic drinks and non-alcoholic, or soft, drinks.

Non-alcoholic drinks include fruit juices, fizzy drinks, squashes, water, milk, tea and coffee.

Alcoholic drinks include wine, beer, cider, sherry and spirits (like gin, whisky and vodka).

Alcohol is made by chemical changes called fermentation. Fermentation changes, for instance, grape juice into wine and apples into cider.

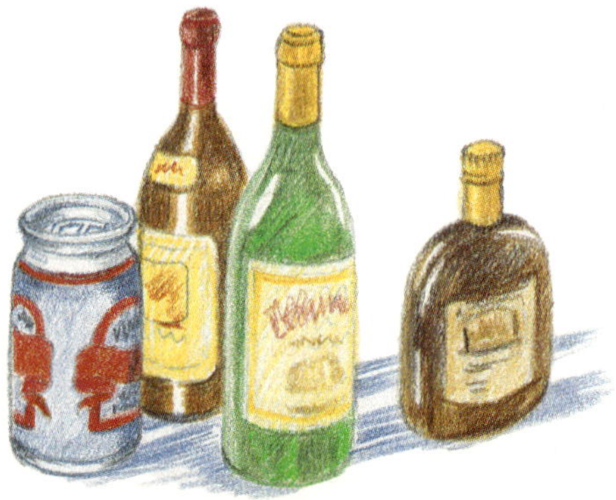

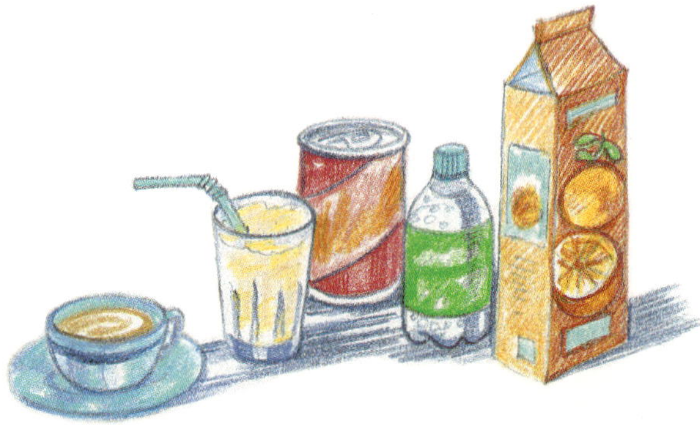

WHAT DOES ALCOHOL DO TO THE BODY?

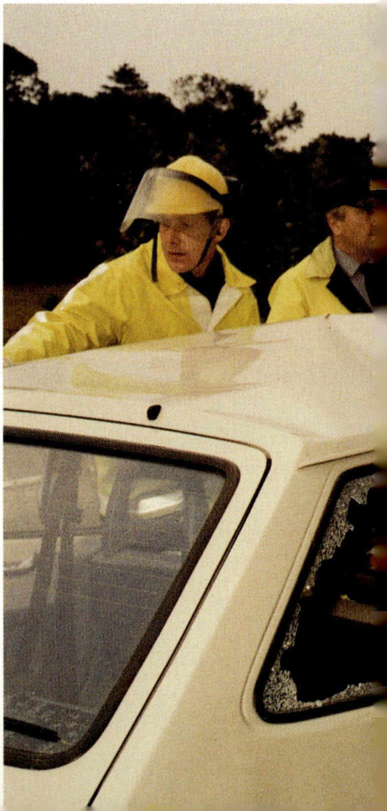

Alcohol slows the body down. In small amounts this can make your body feel more relaxed. But in large amounts it can be very dangerous.

Too much alcohol slows down your brain and this affects the way you move and speak.

Someone who has had too much alcohol may not be able to walk properly and may not be able to speak clearly.

The problem is that people who drink too much often don't realise this. They think that they are walking and talking in the same way as usual.

A drunk person is a danger both to themselves and others.

They cannot look after themselves properly. They may walk off the pavement into the path of a car or, worse, they may think they can drive their car and end up having an accident, injuring or even killing someone.

Too much drink makes some people get angry easily.

The police are often called to help sort out fights in which at least one person is drunk.

It makes some people dizzy or sleepy. They may even fall unconscious. This too can be dangerous.

Your body cannot cope with too much alcohol at one time and so it tries to get rid of it by making you sick it up.

If someone is unconscious he or she could choke and die on their vomit.

Alcohol can be particularly bad for young, growing bodies.

This is part of the reason why young people are not allowed by law to drink alcoholic drinks in pubs until they are 18.

However, too much alcohol for too long, at any age, can lead to brain, liver, kidney or muscle damage.

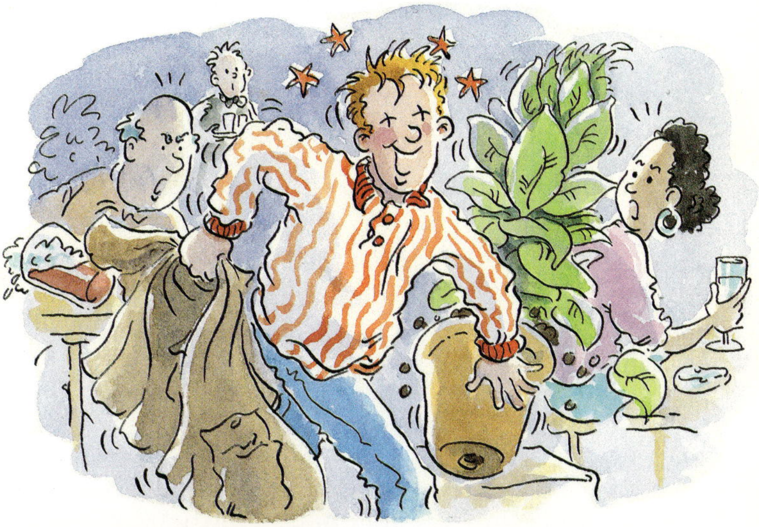

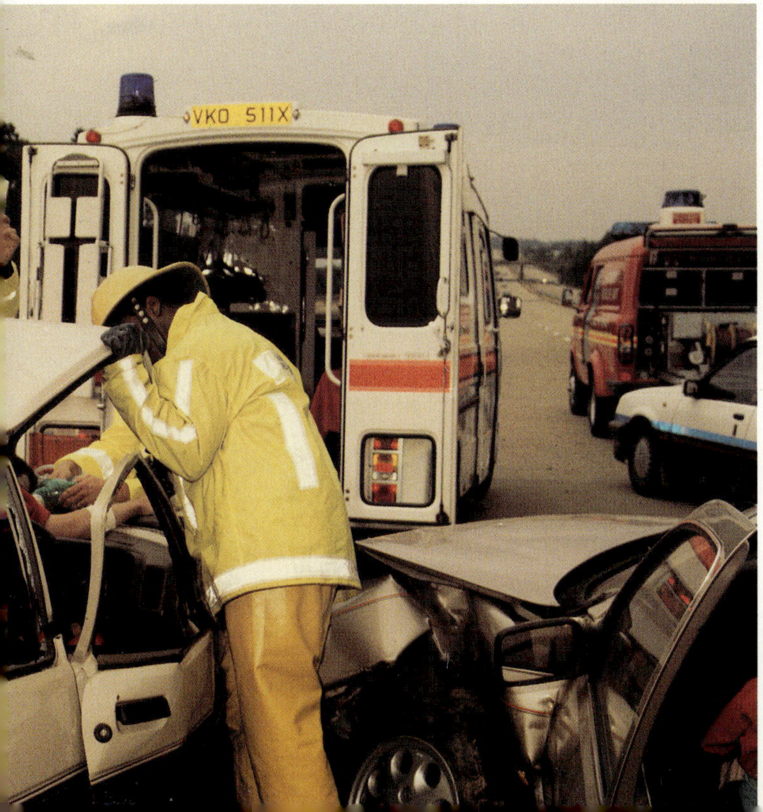

Some religions do not allow their followers of any age to have alcoholic drinks.

But many people in this country and all around the world do enjoy an alcoholic drink.

Some experts say that drinking a small amount of alcohol regularly may help to stop people having heart attacks.

The important thing is to drink it sensibly.

Drugs

At some time as you grow up you will probably be offered drugs.

Knowing something about drugs, and the harmful effects they can have on people, will be useful if you are trying to explain why you will not take them.

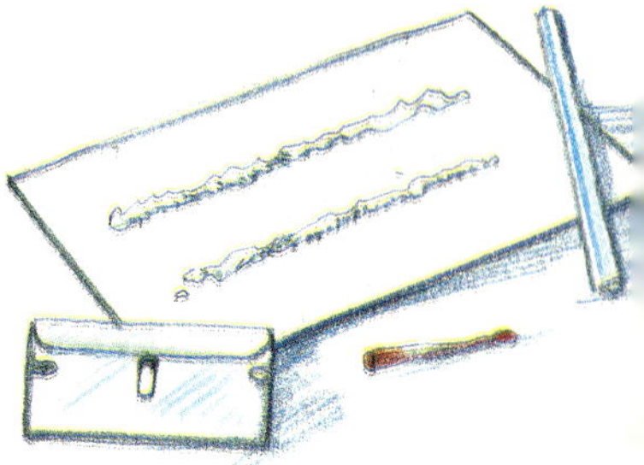

WHY DO PEOPLE TAKE DRUGS?

People often say they take drugs because they like the effects they have. But these effects can be very dangerous.

Without drugs you have control over your body and mind. You are in charge. But when people take drugs they may find that they lose that control and instead of being in charge of their own bodies, the drugs are in charge. This can feel very frightening. It can also be dangerous.

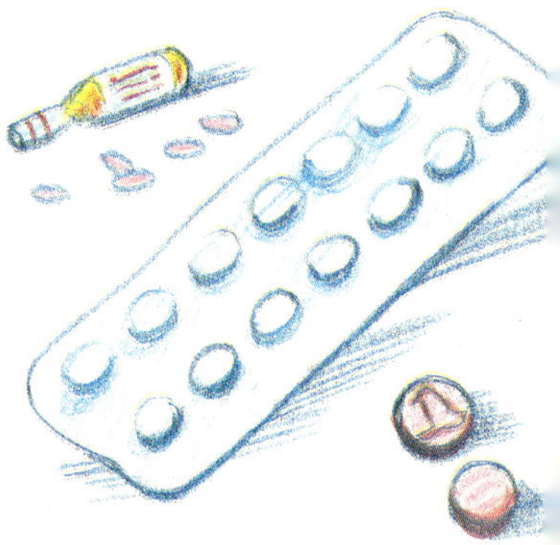

People sometimes take terrible risks when they have taken drugs.

They may think they can do things that they can't or things that are unsafe or even impossible. People have died thinking that they could fly or swim across a river.

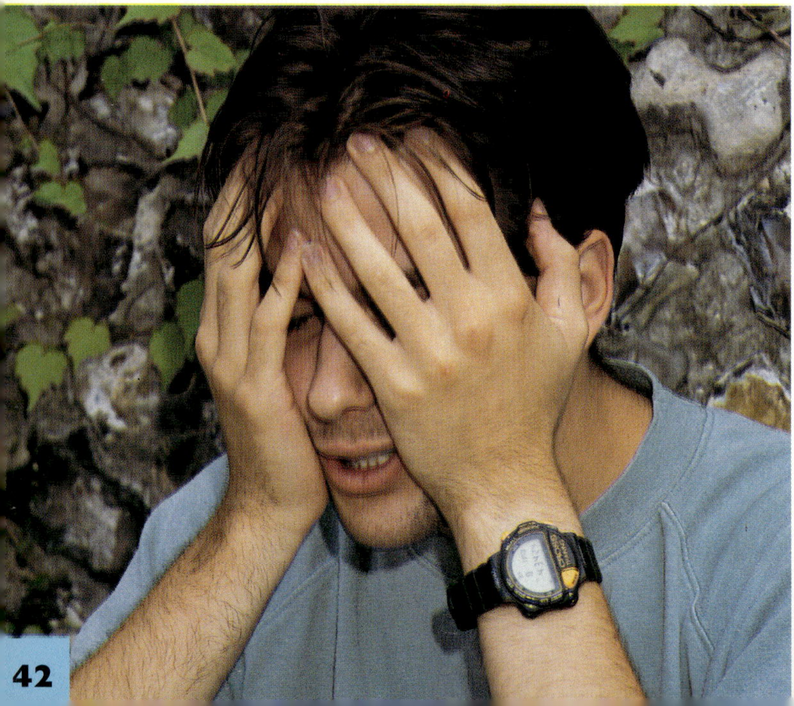

Some of the main drugs are cocaine, heroin, amphetamines, LSD, ecstasy and cannabis.

But drugs have lots of slang names too like trips, blow, smack and whizz.

Drugs like these are illegal. That means that it is against the law to have them.

Some are addictive which means that the body starts to need the drugs even though they are bad for it.

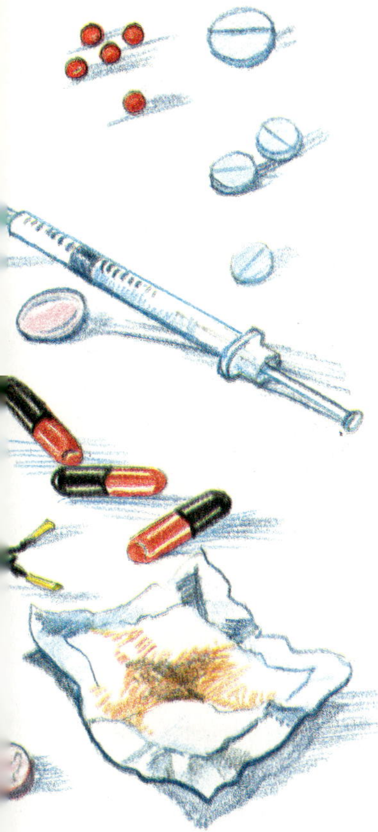

SOLVENT MISUSE OR 'SNIFFING'

The phrase 'solvent misuse' covers lots of different things.

It includes sniffing glue, the gas in cigarette lighter refill canisters and aerosols.

It has the same sort of effect as getting drunk but is much more dangerous.

It isn't just that you lose control of your body but that it can also make your heart beat too fast. It can even give you a heart attack and kill you instantly.

At least two people a week die from solvent misuse.

One in every three of these people was sniffing for the first time.

They probably thought that it wouldn't hurt just to try it once. But for them it was one time too many.

Different drugs are taken in different ways.

They can be swallowed, smoked, sniffed or injected.

Some are pills, some are on little tabs of paper, some are powders, some look like the tobacco in cigarettes.

MEDICINES

Drugs aren't always dangerous and illegal. Some drugs, like those from a doctor, are used as medicines.

These can be good for you and make you well if you are ill.

But even these have to be used carefully.

You should always take the amount that you are told to take. Never take any more than this, or use medicine belonging to anyone else.

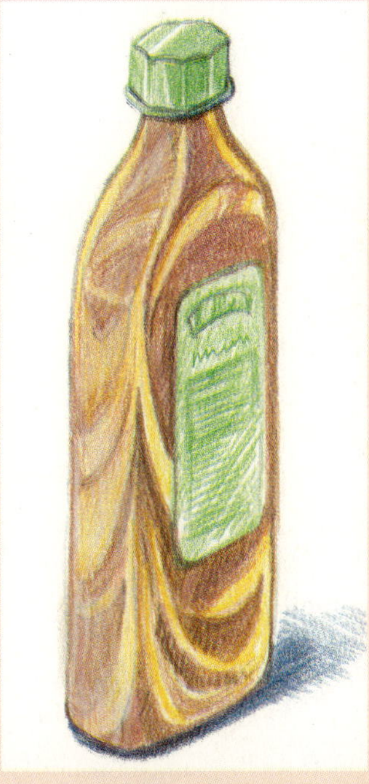

Independence

Part of growing up is about learning to be independent. That is, to think more for yourself and to stand on your own two feet.

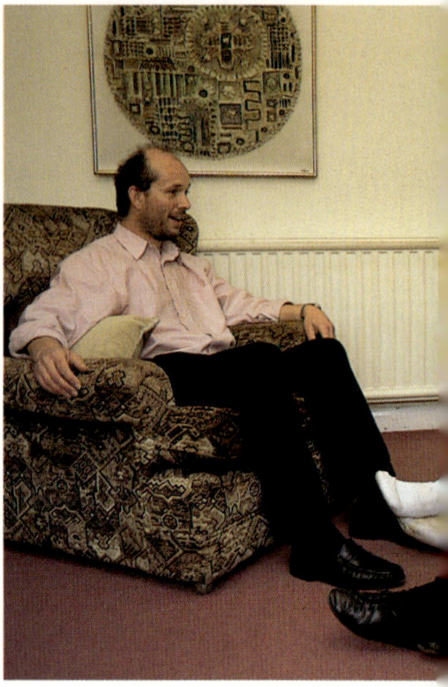

But, in the same way that your body does not change from a child's to an adult's overnight, so becoming independent takes time too.

You will probably start to have your own views about things and you may want to begin to make choices for yourself.

At first, parents sometimes find it difficult to get used to this. It can lead to arguments. For instance, perhaps there's something on television on a Friday evening that goes on quite late but that you desperately want to watch.

Your parents say no.

You think they are being mean.

They think you aren't being fair.

And you all end up having an argument.

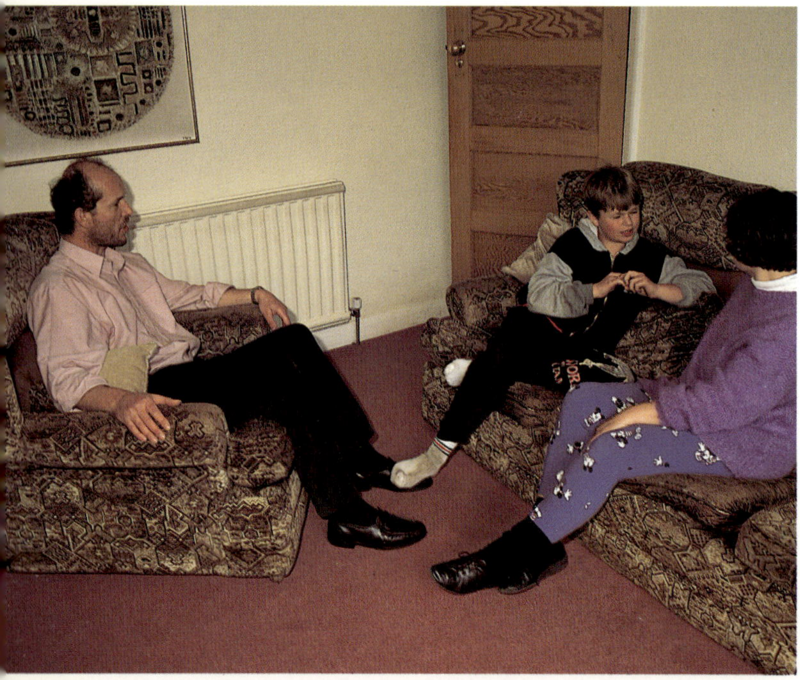

Many arguments like this can be avoided.

Showing your parents that you have thought about the problem might help.

Saying that you know it is on late but that it is a Friday night and that there is no school in the morning, that you could go to bed earlier the next night and that it was something you particularly wanted to watch, might make your parents more likely to agree to it.

Being angry or sulky about something you want to do but aren't allowed to is unlikely to help the situation.

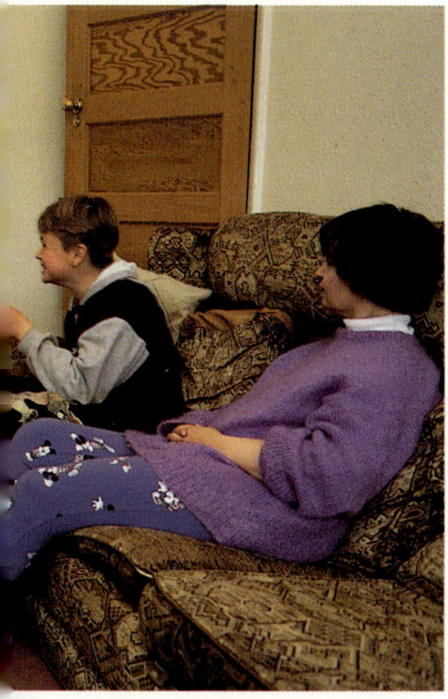

If your parents let you go to a friend's house on condition that you are back home by a particular time, make sure that you are back by then. Or, at least, ring up to let them know what is happening.

If you don't, you only have yourself to blame if they refuse to let you go again.

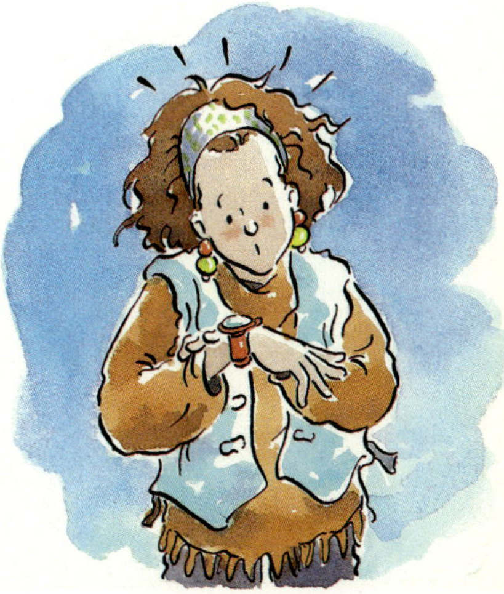

Being independent means being free to make up your own mind about things but it also means that you can't blame other people for the results of those choices.

A proper discussion with a bit of give and take is much more likely to keep everyone happy.

Parents aren't usually just being mean when they refuse to allow you to do something.

Most parents are only concerned for you. As you grow up you will probably start to want to do things on your own. They are bound to worry about you.

The best way to make them worry less is to show them that you can make sensible decisions and that they can trust you to do what you say.

So, growing up isn't just about having a changing body. Growing up has a lot to do with the way you live your life, too.

It can be a confusing time. It is also an exciting time.

Are you ready for the adventure?

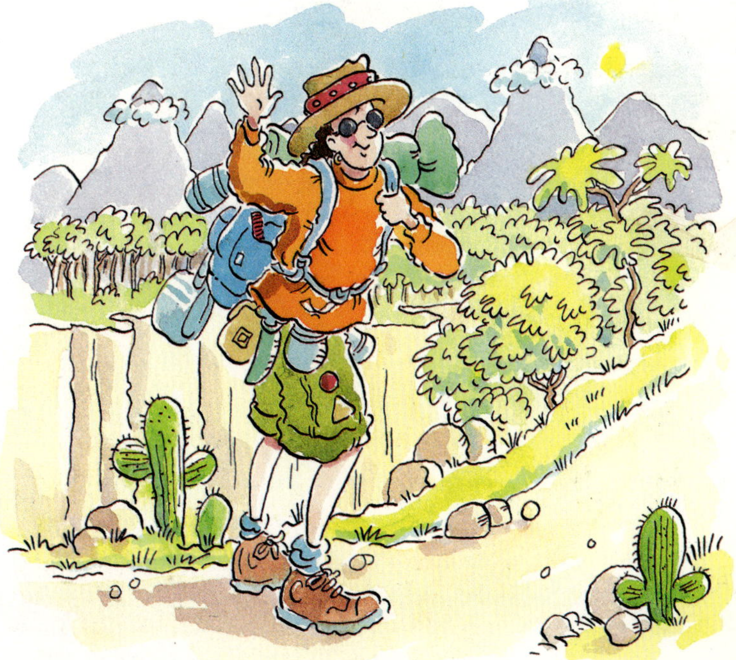

Glossary

addiction	a habit, for example drug-taking, that it is impossible to break.
adolescence	the time between being a child and an adult.
AIDS	a group of illnesses caused by a virus which weakens the body's immune system.
amniotic sac	the bag of fluid that a baby develops in.
areola	the dark circle around the nipple.
carbon monoxide	a poisonous, colourless gas.
contraception	ways of preventing a baby being made.
ejaculation	when semen squirts out of a penis.
embryo	the name given to a developing baby for about the first eight weeks.
fallopian tubes	the tubes that egg cells travel along to the uterus.
family planning	contraception and advice about contraception.
genitals	the parts of the body that are between the legs – the sex organs.
HIV	the short name for the virus called the Human Immuno-deficiency Virus.
hormones	chemicals that are made by the body.
independence	being able to think and act for yourself without being dependent on anyone else.
nicotine	a poisonous substance found in tobacco.
ovaries	where a woman's egg cells are produced.
puberty	the time when the body is gradually changing from child to adult and becoming able to make babies.
sexually transmitted diseases	diseases that are caught after having sex with an infected person.
solvent misuse	inhaling (or 'sniffing') substances such as lighter fuel, glue or aerosols.

OTHER BOOKS TO READ

Growing Up by Susan Meredith (Usborne, 1996)

Babies by Robyn Gee (Usborne, 1996)

The Facts of Life by Susan Meredith and Robyn Gee (Usborne, 1996)

Growing Up by Karen Bryant-Mole (Wayland, 1994)

We're talking about AIDS by Karen Bryant-Mole (Wayland, 1994)

We're talking about Smoking by Karen Bryant-Mole (Wayland, 1995)

We're talking about Drugs by Jenny Bryan (Wayland, 1995)

Index